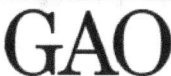

I0425942

May 2012

MEDICARE

Review of the First Year of CMS's Durable Medical Equipment Competitive Bidding Program's Round 1 Rebid

To access this report electronically, scan this QR Code.

Don't have a QR code reader? Several are available for free online.

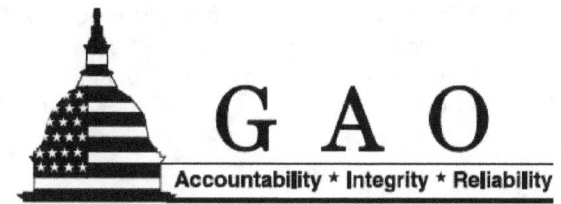

GAO Accountability ★ Integrity ★ Reliability

GAO-12-693

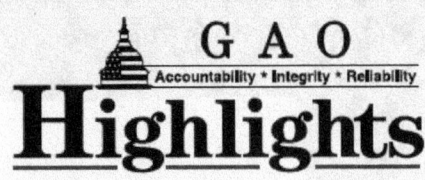

Highlights of GAO-12-693, a report to congressional committees

MEDICARE

Review of the First Year of CMS's Durable Medical Equipment Competitive Bidding Program's Round 1 Rebid

Why GAO Did This Study

To achieve Medicare savings for DME, the Medicare Prescription Drug, Improvement, and Modernization Act of 2003 (MMA) required that CMS implement the CBP for certain DME. In 2008, the Medicare Improvements for Patients and Providers Act (MIPPA) terminated the first round of supplier contracts and required CMS to repeat the CBP round 1—referred to as the round 1 rebid, resulting in the award of contracts to suppliers with payments that began January 1, 2011. CMS has estimated that the rebid will lead to significant savings for Medicare.

MIPPA requires GAO to examine certain aspects of the CBP. In this report, GAO reviews (1) the outcomes of the CBP round 1 rebid process; (2) the effect of the CBP round 1 rebid on DME suppliers; (3) how the CBP round 1 rebid has affected Medicare beneficiary access to and satisfaction with selected DME; and (4) the extent to which the CBP round 1 rebid has affected the utilization of selected DME items.

To examine CBP outcomes and effects, GAO analyzed data from CMS and its feedback provided to bidding suppliers, analyzed 2011 CBP data about different types of suppliers, and interviewed CMS and CBP contractor officials, DME industry groups, and suppliers. To examine CBP's effects on beneficiary access, GAO analyzed Medicare claims data for the first six months of 2011 because the data for those months were the most complete, and compared it to the same months in 2010.

View GAO-12-693. For more information, contact Kathleen M. King at (202) 512-7114 or kingk@gao.gov.

What GAO Found

The Centers for Medicare and Medicaid Services (CMS), within the Department of Health and Human Services (HHS), implemented the durable medical equipment (DME) competitive bidding program's (CBP) bidding process for the round 1 rebid. Nearly the same number of suppliers submitted a similar number of bids for both the CBP round 1 rebid and round 1. Many suppliers continued to have difficulty complying with financial documentation requirements; however, the number of bids disqualified in the round 1 rebid was significantly less than for round 1. After being notified of their bid results, some suppliers were found to have bids that were disqualified incorrectly and were subsequently offered round 1 rebid contracts. About one-third of the bidding suppliers were awarded CBP contracts.

Relatively few CBP contract suppliers (those awarded CBP contracts) had their contracts terminated by CMS, voluntarily canceled their contracts, or were involved in ownership changes. Under the CBP, non-contract suppliers (those not awarded CBP contracts) can grandfather certain rental DME for beneficiaries they were servicing prior to the implementation of CBP until CBP-covered beneficiaries' rental periods expire. Also, some CBP contract suppliers entered into subcontracting agreements with non-contract suppliers to furnish certain services to CBP-covered beneficiaries in the round 1 rebid.

CMS's ongoing multiple monitoring activities generally indicate that beneficiary DME access and satisfaction have not been affected by CBP. Although some of these efforts have limitations, in the aggregate, they provide useful information to CMS regarding beneficiary access and satisfaction.

Early data indicate that utilization has decreased in some CBP-covered DME categories. GAO's review of Medicare claims data found that fewer beneficiaries in competitive bidding areas received some CBP-covered items in any of the first six months of 2011 than in the same month of 2010.

Although the first year of the CBP round 1 rebid has been completed, it is too soon to determine its full effects on Medicare beneficiaries and DME suppliers. GAO found that, in general, the round 1 rebid was successfully implemented. GAO also found that utilization of selected DME declined in the CBP areas; while there are many possible reasons for this, it does not necessarily indicate that beneficiaries have not had access to needed DME. GAO does not assume that all pre-CBP utilization was appropriate and the CBP may have reduced unnecessary utilization of DME. More experience with DME competitive bidding is needed, particularly to see if evidence of beneficiary access problems emerges. For that reason, it is important to continue monitoring changes in the number of suppliers serving CBP-covered beneficiaries.

In commenting on a draft of this report, HHS noted that the CBP round 1 rebid resulted in savings of more than $200 million in its first year. HHS also cited the results of CMS's monitoring of beneficiaries' access to DME in CBP areas as evidence that the CBP did not affect beneficiaries adversely.

Contents

Figures

Abbreviations

CBP	competitive bidding program
CMS	Centers for Medicare & Medicaid Services
CAO	competitive acquisition ombudsman
CPAP/RAD	continuous positive airway pressure devices and respiratory assist devices
CSR	customer service representative
DBidS	Durable Medical Equipment, Prosthetics, Orthotics, and Supplies Bidding System
DME	durable medical equipment
DMEPOS	durable medical equipment, prosthetics, orthotics, and supplies
HCPCS	Healthcare Common Procedure Coding System
HHS	Department of Health and Human Services
MIPPA	Medicare Improvements for Patients and Providers Act of 2008
MMA	Medicare Prescription Drug, Improvement, and Modernization Act of 2003
NSC	National Supplier Clearinghouse
NF	nursing facilities
OIG	Office of Inspector General
PAOC	Program Advisory and Oversight Committee
PTAN	provider transaction access number
SNF	skilled nursing facilities

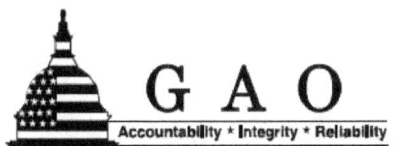

United States Government Accountability Office
Washington, DC 20548

May 9, 2012

The Honorable Max Baucus
Chairman
The Honorable Orrin Hatch
Ranking Member
Committee on Finance
United States Senate

The Honorable Fred Upton
Chairman
The Honorable Henry Waxman
Ranking Member
Committee on Energy and Commerce
House of Representatives

The Honorable Dave Camp
Chairman
The Honorable Sander Levin
Ranking Member
Committee on Ways and Means
House of Representatives

In 2010, Medicare—a federal health insurance program[1]—spent
$8.1 billion on durable medical equipment (DME), prosthetics, orthotics,
and related supplies for beneficiaries.[2] The Medicare program is
administered by the Centers for Medicare and Medicaid (CMS) within the

---

[1]Medicare is for people age 65 and older, individuals under age 65 with certain disabilities,
and individuals diagnosed with end-stage renal disease.

[2]DME is equipment that serves a medical purpose, can withstand repeated use, is
generally not useful in the absence of an illness or injury, and is appropriate for use in the
home including, for example, wheelchairs and hospital beds. Prosthetic devices (other
than dental) are defined as devices needed to replace body parts or functions such as
artificial limbs, enteral nutrition, and cardiac pacemakers. Orthotic devices are defined as
providing rigid or semi-rigid support for weak or deformed body parts or restricting or
eliminating motion in a diseased or injured part of the body, such as leg, arm, back, and
neck braces. Medicare-reimbursed supplies are items that are used and consumed with
DME, such as drugs used for inhalation therapy, or that need to be replaced frequently
(usually daily), such as surgical dressings. Collectively DME, prosthetics, and orthotics are
referred to as DMEPOS. For this report, the term DME refers to all DMEPOS items
included in the CBP.

Department of Health and Human Services (HHS). Most Medicare beneficiaries participate in Medicare Part B,[3] which helps pay for DMEPOS items and supplies, such as oxygen, wheelchairs, hospital beds, walkers, orthotics, prosthetics, and supplies if they are medically necessary and prescribed by a physician. Medicare beneficiaries typically obtain DMEPOS items from suppliers, which submit claims for payment to Medicare on behalf of beneficiaries. Both we and the HHS Office of Inspector General (OIG) have reported that Medicare and its beneficiaries have sometimes paid higher-than-market rates for various medical equipment and supply items.[4] These overpayments increase costs to both Medicare and its beneficiaries.

To achieve Medicare savings for DMEPOS and to address DMEPOS fraud concerns, Congress, through the Medicare Prescription Drug, Improvement, and Modernization Act of 2003 (MMA),[5] required CMS to phase in a competitive bidding program (CBP). Under CBP, DME suppliers are competitively selected to furnish certain DME product

---

[3]Medicare Part B helps pay for certain physician, outpatient hospital, laboratory, and other services, and medical equipment and supplies—DMEPOS. Beneficiaries are required to pay a monthly premium for Part B coverage, an annual deductible, and coinsurance. In general, Medicare beneficiaries pay 20 percent—the coinsurance—of the Medicare fee schedule payment rate for the DMEPOS item after reaching their annual Medicare Part B deductible. In 2010, CMs reported that Medicare Part B and beneficiaries paid approximately $14.3 billion for DMEPOS.

[4]GAO, *Medicare: CMS Has Addressed Some Implementation Problems from Round 1 of the Durable Medical Equipment Competitive Bidding Program for the Round 1 Rebid*, GAO-10-1057T (Washington, D.C.: Sept. 15, 2010); *Medicare: CMS Working to Address Problems from Round 1 of the Durable Medical Equipment Competitive Bidding Program*, GAO-10-27 (Washington, D.C.: Nov. 6, 2009); *Medicare: Competitive Bidding for Medical Equipment and Supplies Could Reduce Program Payments, but Adequate Oversight Is Critical*, GAO-08-767T (Washington, D.C.: May 6, 2008); *Medicare: Past Experience Can Guide Future Competitive Bidding for Medical Equipment and Supplies*, GAO-04-765 (Washington, D.C.: Sept. 7, 2004); Department of Health and Human Services Office of Inspector General, *A Comparison of Prices for Power Wheelchairs in the Medicare Program*, OEI-03-03-00460 (Washington, D.C.: April 2004); and Janet Rehnquist, Inspector General, Department of Health and Human Services, *Medicare Reimbursement for Medical Equipment and Supplies*, testimony before the Senate Committee on Appropriations, Subcommittee on Labor, Health and Human Services, and Education, 107th Cong., 2nd sess., June 12, 2002.

[5]Medicare Prescription Drug, Improvement, and Modernization Act of 2003, Pub. L. No. 108-173, § 302(b), 117 Stat. 2066, 2224-30 (2003) (codified as amended at 42 U.S.C. § 1395w-3).

categories[6] to Medicare beneficiaries in designated competitive bidding areas.[7] On January 1, 2011, CMS began operating the CBP—referred to as the CBP round 1 rebid—in nine competitive bidding areas[8] for selected DME items in nine product categories.[9] The DME suppliers that won CBP contracts—contract suppliers—are paid at the competitively determined payments for the CBP-covered DME items[10] which must be less than or equal to Medicare's fee schedule[11] payments for the same items. Of the estimated 47 million Medicare beneficiaries, about 2 million CBP-covered beneficiaries reside in the nine competitive bidding areas.[12]

---

[6]A product category is a grouping of related items used to treat a similar medical condition.

[7]A competitive bidding area is either a metropolitan statistical area or a part thereof. Metropolitan statistical areas are designated by the Office of Management and Budget and include major cities and the suburban areas surrounding them.

[8]The nine CBP round 1 rebid competitive bidding areas are: Charlotte (Charlotte-Gastonia-Concord, North Carolina and South Carolina); Cincinnati (Cincinnati-Middletown, Ohio, Kentucky, and Indiana); Cleveland (Cleveland-Elyria-Mentor, Ohio); Dallas (Dallas-Fort Worth-Arlington, Texas); Kansas City (Kansas City, Missouri and Kansas); Miami (Miami-Fort Lauderdale-Pompano Beach, Florida); Orlando (Orlando-Kissimmee, Florida); Pittsburgh (Pittsburgh, Pennsylvania); and Riverside (Riverside-San Bernardino-Ontario, California).

[9]The CBP round 1 rebid's nine product categories are: complex power wheelchairs (complex rehabilitative power wheelchairs and related accessories—limited to group 2—power wheelchairs with power options); CPAP/RAD (continuous positive airway pressure devices, respiratory assist devices, and related supplies and accessories); enteral (enteral nutrients, equipment, and supplies); hospital beds (hospital beds and related accessories); mail-order diabetic supplies; oxygen (oxygen supplies and equipment); standard power wheelchairs (standard power wheelchairs, scooters, and related accessories); walkers (walkers and related accessories); and support surfaces (support surfaces limited to group 2 mattresses and overlays—pressure reducing support surfaces for persons with or at high risk for pressure ulcers—in the Miami competitive bidding area only.)

[10]The terms CBP-covered items and CBP-covered beneficiaries are used since not all Medicare-covered DME items are included in the CBP and not all beneficiaries residing in a CBP competitive bidding area are covered by CBP.

[11]In general, DME fee schedule rates are subject to national floor and ceiling limits, and may be updated by the consumer price index for all urban consumers. Medicare payment for DME is generally equal to 80 percent of the lesser of either the supplier's actual charge or the Medicare fee schedule for a particular item or service.

[12]Beneficiaries who reside in the CBP competitive bidding areas and are enrolled in Medicare Advantage health plans, which are operated by private companies, are not subject to CBP.

CMS began implementing CBP in 2007 and 2008—referred to as round 1.[13] However, the Medicare Improvements for Patient and Providers Act of 2008 (MIPPA)[14] terminated the CBP round 1 supplier contracts on July 15, 2008, and required CMS to repeat the CBP round 1—referred to as the round 1 rebid. To compensate for the loss of the projected Medicare savings due to the termination of CBP round 1 and delay of CBP and to ensure budget neutrality, MIPPA reduced the Medicare payments for the DME items that had been included in round 1 by 9.5 percent nationally.[15] In 2009, CMS began the CBP round 1 rebid bidding process, and in January 2011, the CBP round 1 rebid began.

MIPPA requires us to examine particular issues regarding early results from the ongoing CBP round 1 rebid.[16] In this report, we review (1) the outcomes of the CBP round 1 rebid process including bid disqualifications and contracts awarded; (2) the effect of the CBP round 1 rebid on DME suppliers; (3) how the CBP round 1 rebid has affected Medicare beneficiary access to and satisfaction with selected DME; (4) the extent to which the CBP round 1 rebid has affected the utilization of selected DME items; and (5) the costs for CMS to implement, and for DME suppliers to participate, in CBP.

To examine the outcomes of the CBP round 1 rebid, we analyzed data from CMS and reviewed feedback that CMS provided to suppliers to explain bid deficiencies. We also reviewed CMS's notification to suppliers that did not win a contract describing the opportunity to have their bids reviewed. To examine the effect of the CBP round 1 rebid on DME suppliers, we analyzed 2011 CMS data on contract suppliers including those that were terminated by CMS or voluntarily withdrew from CBP, grandfathered suppliers, subcontracting suppliers, and suppliers' ownership changes, and interviewed CMS and CBP contractor officials, DME industry groups, and selected suppliers.

---

[13]CMS conducted demonstrations from 1999 to 2002 that showed that DME competitive bidding would save money for both the Medicare program and for Medicare beneficiaries in lower coinsurance.

[14]Pub. L. No. 110-275, § 154(a)(1), 122 Stat. 2494, 2560-3 (2008) (codified, as amended, at 42 U.S.C. § 1395w-3).

[15]Pub. L. No. 110-275, § 154(a)(2), 122 Stat. at 2563 (2008) (codified, as amended, at 42 U.S.C. § 1395m(a)(14)).

[16]Pub. L. No. 110-275, § 154(c), 122 Stat. at 2565-6.

To examine how the CBP round 1 rebid has affected Medicare beneficiary access to and satisfaction with selected DME items, we analyzed 2011 CMS data, including CBP inquiry data from the 1-800-MEDICARE beneficiary help line, CBP complaint data, and interviewed CMS and CBP contractor officials and Medicare beneficiary advocacy groups. To examine the extent to which the CBP round 1 rebid has affected the beneficiary utilization of certain DME items, we obtained and analyzed the first six months of Medicare claims data both pre-CBP (2010) and post-CBP (2011) because data for those months are the most complete. We used these data to determine whether the number of CBP-covered beneficiaries utilizing CBP-covered items and services increased or decreased in the first 6 months of 2011 when the CBP round 1 began compared to the same time period in 2010. We compared the number of Medicare beneficiaries using selected CBP-covered items—chosen by CMS as the top 80 percent highest cost and highest utilization items—in the nine competitive bidding areas to non-competitive bidding areas (see appendix I for the DME items included in our analysis).[17] In submitting claims for Medicare payments, suppliers use a standardized coding system—the Healthcare Common Procedure Coding System (HCPCS). Since HCPCS codes identify a category of like DMEPOS items, for example, hospital beds, individual HCPCS codes can include a broad range of items that serve the same general purpose but that vary in price and characteristics and do not identify an item's manufacturer, or brand or trade name, we determined that an analysis to compare utilization of items included in the same HCPCS code would not be meaningful.

To describe the costs for CMS to implement and for DME suppliers to participate in CBP, we reported the CBP round 1 rebid pre-implementation costs provided to us by CMS. We also interviewed CMS officials, DME supplier trade groups, and selected DME suppliers to obtain descriptions and estimates of CBP-related administrative costs and suppliers' participation expenses.

To assess the reliability for all the data we received from CMS, we reviewed and identified outliers in data, and interviewed CMS and other appropriate officials to clarify and resolve any discrepancies. We

---

[17]Contract suppliers submit the HCPCS codes for the CBP-covered items they plan to furnish each quarter to CMS through the Palmetto GBA website https://www.dmecompetitivebid.com/secure/cbicsecure.nsf/FormC, which also provides a listing by product category of the top HCPCS codes.

assessed the reliability of the Medicare claims data from the 100 Percent Standard Analytic Files from CMS by reviewing existing information about the data and the systems that produced them, performing appropriate electronic data checks, and interviewing individuals from CMS, CMS's Pricing, Data Analysis and Coding Contractor, and two DME Medicare Administrative Contractors. We determined that these data were sufficiently reliable for the purposes of this report.

Our findings are based on the limited evidence available at the time we did our work, and more data will become available as CBP continues. We conducted this performance audit from May 2011 through May 2012 in accordance with generally accepted government auditing standards. Those standards require that we plan and perform the audit to obtain sufficient, appropriate evidence to provide a reasonable basis for our findings based on our audit objectives. We believe that the evidence obtained provides a reasonable basis for our findings based on our audit objectives.

Background

Medicare Payments

Medicare pays for most DMEPOS through fee schedules based on suppliers' previous charges to Medicare.[18] The fee schedule payment is generally equal to 80 percent of the lesser of either the supplier's actual charge or the Medicare fee schedule for a particular item or service. In general, Medicare beneficiaries are responsible for paying the supplier the remaining 20 percent—the coinsurance.[19] To process all Medicare

---

[18]Medicare adjusts fee schedules for DMEPOS for each state, reflecting geographic price differences that are subject to national floor and ceiling limits. The applicable state fee schedule is determined by the Medicare beneficiary's residence, not the supplier's location.

[19]For suppliers, Medicare assignment—accepting Medicare's reimbursement amount for an item as payment in full and limiting the amount the beneficiary can be billed for that item—is optional. If a supplier agrees to assignment, then Medicare generally pays 80 percent of the amount to the supplier and the Medicare beneficiary is responsible for paying the supplier the remaining 20 percent—referred to as the coinsurance payment, once the beneficiary's annual deductible has been met. If the supplier does not accept assignment, the supplier is not limited to charging the beneficiary 20 percent of the Medicare reimbursement for that item or service and the beneficiary can be billed for whatever balance is due. For CBP-covered items, Medicare assignment is mandatory for suppliers.

DMEPOS payment claims including coverage and payment determinations, CMS contracts with four DME Medicare Administrative Contractors.

The CBP

CMS and its CBP implementation contractor—Palmetto GBA—administer and implement CBP and its bidding rounds. To be eligible to submit bids to furnish CBP-covered DME items in one or more product categories in one or more of the competitive bidding areas, suppliers must first meet several requirements. Specifically, suppliers must have an active National Supplier Clearinghouse (NSC)[20] number that makes them eligible to bill Medicare for DME, have met Medicare enrollment and quality standards,[21] have a surety bond,[22] and be accredited. After the bid window closes, Palmetto GBA reviews bids to determine whether each supplier's bid submission is complete and compliant with the bidding requirements, and whether the supplier's financial score[23] meets CMS's minimum financial standard threshold to be eligible to compete on price. If the bid meets these requirements, it is considered a qualified bid and can then compete on price. Before comparing prices, Palmetto GBA reviews each qualified bid's estimated capacity projections—the supplier's anticipated ability to provide the volume of items claimed in the bid in light of the supplier's historical capacity, expansion plans, and financial score.

[20]The National Supplier Clearinghouse is the CMS contractor responsible for processing Medicare enrollment applications for DMEPOS suppliers and may revoke a supplier's enrollment if, for example, a supplier loses its Medicare accreditation. Beginning in 2012, CMS has a new contractor to conduct automated screening of Medicare enrollment for all providers and suppliers including DMEPOS suppliers. CMS also has a new contractor to conduct site visits to ensure that enrolled suppliers have a physical facility on an appropriate site, but the NSC continues to conduct site visits for DMEPOS suppliers.

[21]For a list of Medicare enrollment standards applying to all DMEPOS suppliers, see 42 C.F.R. § 424.57(c). For a list of Medicare quality standards applying to all DMEPOS suppliers, see https://www.cms.gov/medicareprovidersupenroll/10_DMEPOS supplierstandards.asp (accessed on April 20, 2012).

[22]Certain DMEPOS suppliers are required to post a $50,000 surety bond for each business location. Surety bonds are designed to reduce the amount of money that is lost due to fraudulent or abusive billing schemes by suppliers.

[23]The financial score is used to determine a supplier's financial viability and is calculated using the bidding supplier's credit score and 10 financial measures that CMS describes as standard accounting measures.

Palmetto GBA uses several steps to compare prices and identify the winning bids.[24] First, Palmetto GBA reviews the DME bid item prices submitted by suppliers with qualified bids and uses a methodology to calculate what is known as a composite bid to allow for a comparison of prices submitted across bidding suppliers with qualified bids. A composite bid is determined by summing all of the weights assigned to each item in a product category—with each item weight calculated using national beneficiary utilization data for that item compared to the other items within that product category. Once the composite price has been calculated, the bids are ordered by the lowest to highest composite bid price in each product category in each competitive bidding area. When the bids have been ordered, Palmetto GBA calculates the cumulative projected capacity of the competing bids—which indicates the capacity that each supplier projects it could furnish throughout an entire competitive bidding area each year. Palmetto GBA begins with the lowest composite price and moves up the ordered list to identify the bid where the suppliers' cumulative projected capacity meets or exceeds CMS's estimated beneficiary demand, which is referred to as the pivotal bid. Although many bids can be qualified to compete on price, only those with composite prices that are equal to or less than the pivotal bid are determined to be winning suppliers, based on price, and are used to establish Medicare's CBP single payment amounts for each item in a product category in a competitive bidding area. Specifically, for each item, the winning bids' price offers are ordered from lowest to highest and the median bid price offered by these suppliers for that item becomes the single payment amount. To ensure there is a sufficient number of suppliers and to meet its target goal of awarding at least five contracts in each product category in each competitive bidding area,[25] CMS caps the estimated projected capacity of any single supplier to 20 percent of the total projected beneficiary demand for each product category in each

---

[24]For a figure indicating the CBP process steps used to identify winning bids, see page 10 of GAO-10-27.

[25]If there are five suppliers with qualified bids, CMS will award at least five contracts in each product category in each competitive bidding area. If there are less than five suppliers with qualified bids, CMS must award contracts to at least two suppliers if the suppliers have sufficient capacity to satisfy beneficiary demand in the product category in the competitive bidding area.

competitive bidding area, regardless of the capacity estimated by the supplier in its bid.[26]

The CBP single payment amounts are required to be less than or equal to the Medicare fee-for-service payments for the same items.[27] The same DME item may have a different CBP single payment amount in each competitive bidding area. CMS offers the winning suppliers 3-year contracts to furnish items in the product categories and competitive bidding areas in which they won.[28] All contract suppliers that accept the contract offers must maintain their Medicare billing privileges, state licensure, and accreditation throughout the contract period and accept assignment on all DME items under their contracts.[29] CMS is required, under federal law, to conduct another bidding round to select contract suppliers no less often than once every three years.

CBP Round 1

CBP round 1 was conducted in 2007 and 2008 for 10 competitive bidding areas.[30] For the bidding, CMS chose certain DME items in 10 product categories—generally high-cost and high-volume items and services—that were most likely to result in Medicare savings if competitively acquired. The round 1 contract suppliers were announced in May 2008. However, round 1's bid submission and contract award processes caused concerns about CMS's CBP implementation. In our November 2009 report, we found problems with the bidding process, including poor timing

---

[26]CMS's cap of a supplier's estimated projected capacity to 20 percent does not limit the number of items a supplier can furnish if awarded a contract and suppliers may be able to furnish more than 20 percent of the beneficiary demand in a product category in a competitive bidding area.

[27]The single payment amount is the median of the winning supplier bids for an individual DME item within each product category in each competitive bidding area. The use of the median in setting an item's single payment amount means that the CBP payment may be less than or more than a particular winning supplier's bid price for the item.

[28]The contract period for the CBP round 1 rebid's mail-order diabetic supplies product category is two years.

[29]Medicare assignment is mandatory for CBP contract suppliers and means that a supplier accepts the CBP single payment amount as payment-in-full from Medicare, and can only bill a beneficiary 20 percent of the payment amount.

[30]To begin the program's national phase-in, the CBP round 1's 10 competitive bidding areas were chosen from the largest metropolitan statistical areas. The competitive bidding areas for round 1 and the round 1 rebid were the same except that round 1 included the San Juan (San Juan-Caguas-Guaynabo, Puerto Rico) area.

and lack of clarity in bid submission information and CMS's inability to inform suppliers of missing financial documentation.[31] We also found that CMS did not provide suppliers with timely and clear bid submission information, used an inadequate electronic bid submission system, and did not have a process to inform bidders of missing financial documentation—42 percent of all submitted bids were disqualified due to incomplete financial documentation. In our report, we recommended that if CMS reviews suppliers' disqualified bids during the round 1 rebid and future rounds, it should notify all suppliers of any such process, give suppliers equal opportunity for such reviews, and clearly indicate how suppliers can request a review.

The enactment of MIPPA stopped CBP round 1 two weeks after it began operating and required CMS to repeat the competition for CBP round 1 in 2009. MIPPA also imposed additional criteria for how CMS should conduct later CBP rounds and expand the CBP to additional areas. In addition, MIPPA required that CMS notify bidding suppliers about any missing financial documentation if the suppliers submitted their documentation within a time period known as the covered document review date.[32] MIPPA also required CMS to create a competitive acquisition ombudsman (CAO) to respond to inquiries and complaints made by DME suppliers and individuals concerning the CBP's application. The CAO can work with Palmetto GBA and its local offices.

CBP Round 1 Rebid

In October 2009, CMS began the CBP round 1 rebid process;[33] its 60-day bid window closed in December 2009. In July 2010, CMS announced the competitively determined DME single payment amounts. On January 1, 2011, CBP began with 356 contract suppliers awarded contracts to

---

[31]See GAO-10-27.

[32]MIPPA provided that this process only applies to the timely submission of financial documentation and does not apply to any determination by CMS as to the accuracy or completeness of the documentation submitted or whether the documents meet applicable requirements.

[33]In the CBP round 1 rebid, the product categories were revised to delete the negative pressure wound therapy category—pumps that apply controlled negative or subatmospheric pressure used to treat ulcers or wounds that have not responded to traditional wound treatment methods—and to exclude group 3 complex rehabilitative power wheelchairs (must meet the highest performance requirements, for example, be able to travel at least 12 miles on a single charge of batteries) from the entire CBP, and to delete San Juan (San Juan-Caguas-Guaynabo, Puerto Rico) as a competitive bidding area.

provide DME items and services in nine DME product categories in nine competitive bidding areas.[34] CMS has stated that the CBP round 1 rebid single payment amounts resulted in an average savings of 42 percent in 2011 compared to 2010 for the same items.

CBP Round 2

In January 2012, CMS began CBP's bidding process for round 2. Round 2 will cover 91 metropolitan statistical areas and CMS has determined the competitive bidding areas within those MSAs. The 60-day round 2 bid window was open from January 30, 2012, to March 30, 2012. CMS intends to announce the round 2 winning contract suppliers in spring 2013, and for the contracts and single payment amounts to become effective July 1, 2013.

Round 2 will operate for 3 years and includes the same product categories as the round 1 rebid except for the addition of the negative pressure wound therapy category, the deletion of the complex power wheelchairs and mail-order diabetic supplies categories, and the expansion of the support surfaces category[35] to all competitive bidding areas. A national mail-order diabetic supplies program[36] competition will be conducted at the same time as round 2, and will require bidding suppliers to demonstrate that their bids cover at least 50 percent, by sales volume, of all types of diabetic testing strips on the market.[37] (See fig. 1 for CBP's legislative history and program implementation time line.)

---

[34]The CBP round 1 rebid 3-year contracts expire on December 31, 2013. On April 17, 2012, CMS announced that it planned to begin the bidding process for the second round of contracts in fall 2012.

[35]Support surfaces are pressure reducing support surfaces for persons with or at high risk for pressure ulcers.

[36]The national mail-order competition includes all 50 states, District of Columbia, Puerto Rico, U.S. Virgin Islands, Guam, and American Samoa.

[37]To indicate the testing strip brands they intend to furnish to meet the 50 percent requirement, bidding suppliers complete a National Mail-Order 50 Percent Compliance form as part of their CBP bid submission.

Figure 1: CBP Timeline, 1997-2013

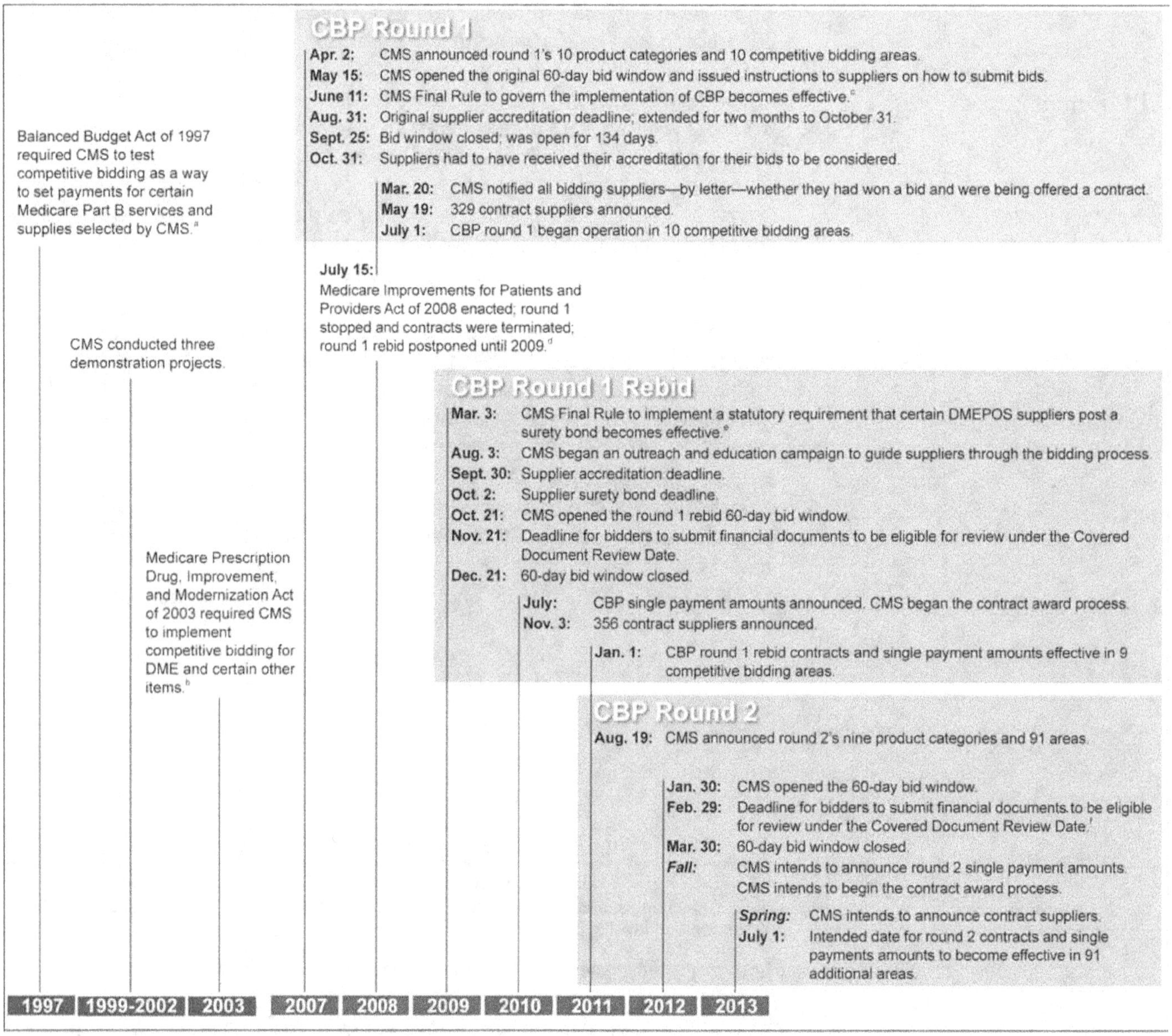

Balanced Budget Act of 1997 required CMS to test competitive bidding as a way to set payments for certain Medicare Part B services and supplies selected by CMS.[a]

CMS conducted three demonstration projects.

Medicare Prescription Drug, Improvement, and Modernization Act of 2003 required CMS to implement competitive bidding for DME and certain other items.[b]

CBP Round 1

Apr. 2:	CMS announced round 1's 10 product categories and 10 competitive bidding areas.
May 15:	CMS opened the original 60-day bid window and issued instructions to suppliers on how to submit bids.
June 11:	CMS Final Rule to govern the implementation of CBP becomes effective.[c]
Aug. 31:	Original supplier accreditation deadline; extended for two months to October 31.
Sept. 25:	Bid window closed; was open for 134 days.
Oct. 31:	Suppliers had to have received their accreditation for their bids to be considered.

Mar. 20:	CMS notified all bidding suppliers—by letter—whether they had won a bid and were being offered a contract.
May 19:	329 contract suppliers announced.
July 1:	CBP round 1 began operation in 10 competitive bidding areas.

July 15:
Medicare Improvements for Patients and Providers Act of 2008 enacted; round 1 stopped and contracts were terminated; round 1 rebid postponed until 2009.[d]

CBP Round 1 Rebid

Mar. 3:	CMS Final Rule to implement a statutory requirement that certain DMEPOS suppliers post a surety bond becomes effective.[e]
Aug. 3:	CMS began an outreach and education campaign to guide suppliers through the bidding process.
Sept. 30:	Supplier accreditation deadline.
Oct. 2:	Supplier surety bond deadline.
Oct. 21:	CMS opened the round 1 rebid 60-day bid window.
Nov. 21:	Deadline for bidders to submit financial documents to be eligible for review under the Covered Document Review Date.
Dec. 21:	60-day bid window closed.

July:	CBP single payment amounts announced. CMS began the contract award process.
Nov. 3:	356 contract suppliers announced.

Jan. 1:	CBP round 1 rebid contracts and single payment amounts effective in 9 competitive bidding areas.

CBP Round 2

Aug. 19:	CMS announced round 2's nine product categories and 91 areas.

Jan. 30:	CMS opened the 60-day bid window.
Feb. 29:	Deadline for bidders to submit financial documents to be eligible for review under the Covered Document Review Date.[f]
Mar. 30:	60-day bid window closed.
Fall:	CMS intends to announce round 2 single payment amounts. CMS intends to begin the contract award process.

Spring:	CMS intends to announce contract suppliers.
July 1:	Intended date for round 2 contracts and single payments amounts to become effective in 91 additional areas.

| 1997 | 1999-2002 | 2003 | 2007 | 2008 | 2009 | 2010 | 2011 | 2012 | 2013 |

Source: GAO analysis of CMS data.

[a]Pub. L. No. 105-33, § 4319(a), 111 Stat. 251, 392-4 (1997) (codified, as amended, at 42 U.S.C. § 1395w-3).

GAO-12-693 DME Competitive Bidding Program

[b]Pub. L. No. 108-173, § 302(b), 117 Stat. 2066, 2224-30 (2003) (codified, as amended, at 42 U.S.C. § 1395w-3). Items and services covered by the competition were DME and related supplies, off-the-shelf orthotics, and enteral nutrients and related equipment and supplies.

[c]CMS, Medicare Program; Competitive Acquisition for Certain Durable Medical Equipment, Prosthetics, Orthotics, and Supplies (DMEPOS) and Other Issues; Final Rule, 72 Fed. Reg. 17,992 (Apr. 10, 2007).

[d]Medicare Improvements for Patients and Providers Act of 2008. Pub. L. No. 110-275, § 154(a)(2), 122 Stat. 2494, 2560-3 (2008) (codified, as amended, at 42 U.S.C. § 1395w-3).

[e]CMS, Medicare Program: Surety Bond Requirement for Suppliers of DMEPOS, Final Rule, 74 Fed. Reg. 166 (Jan. 2, 2009).

[f]CMS must notify suppliers of missing financial documentation if their financial documents are submitted within the covered document review date, which is the later of: (1) 30 days before the final date for the close of the bid window; or (2) 30 days after the bid window opens.

Types of CBP Suppliers

The CBP makes specific provisions for certain types of individual DME suppliers that can bill Medicare. CBP contract suppliers[38] are suppliers that bid and won a CBP contract for at least one product category in at least one competitive bidding area. Non-contract suppliers[39] that do not have a CBP contract may continue to furnish certain DME to beneficiaries in the CBP competitive bidding areas as grandfathered suppliers for existing rental agreements or as subcontractors to contract suppliers.

Small Suppliers and Networks

To ensure that small suppliers are considered when selecting contract suppliers, CMS set a target that 30 percent of the qualified suppliers in each product category in each competitive bidding area are small. CMS defines small suppliers as those that generate gross revenue of $3.5 million or less in annual receipts that include both Medicare and non-Medicare revenue. In cases where the small supplier target goal is not met, CMS can award additional CBP contracts to small suppliers after it determines the number of suppliers needed to meet or exceed CMS's estimated beneficiary demand.

Between 2 to 20 small suppliers are allowed to group together as a network to submit a bid as a single entity under CBP, and to provide services as a contract network if awarded a CBP contract. The suppliers

[38]A contract supplier may be a small or large supplier, a member of a small supplier network, a grandfathering supplier for certain CBP product categories not won, a subcontractor for another contract supplier, or a combination thereof.

[39]A non-contract supplier operating in a competitive bidding area may also be a grandfathering supplier for certain CBP product categories, a subcontractor for another contract supplier, or a combination.

involved must certify that they cannot independently furnish all the competitively bid items in the product category to beneficiaries throughout the entire competitive bidding area for which the network is submitting a bid.

Grandfathered Suppliers

Some suppliers not awarded contracts have the option to choose to continue to furnish certain CBP-covered rental items to beneficiaries who were their customers when CBP began on January 1, 2011, and who are residing in the competitive bidding areas. These suppliers are referred to as grandfathered suppliers.[40] It is the beneficiaries' choice whether to remain with their grandfathered supplier or to select a CBP contract supplier.[41] Many CBP-covered items that are rented can be grandfathered including, for example, oxygen and oxygen equipment,[42] capped rental DME[43]—such as hospital beds—and inexpensive and routinely purchased DME for the remaining rental months.[44] Once the relevant rental periods expire or a beneficiary decides to select a contract supplier, the grandfathered supplier can no longer provide the CBP-covered items and services to the beneficiary.

---

[40]Where a beneficiary permanently resides determines whether they are a CBP-covered beneficiary; a beneficiary's residence is the address used for Social Security.

[41]If a non-contract supplier chooses not to grandfather, or the beneficiary chooses to select a contract supplier, the beneficiary's current and new supplier must coordinate the pick-up and delivery of the affected DME equipment, and CMS requires certain beneficiary notifications be made.

[42]Suppliers that furnished oxygen and oxygen equipment to a beneficiary during the 36th month of continuous use are required to continue to furnish the equipment after the 36 months for any period of medical need during the remainder of the reasonable useful lifetime of the equipment; this obligation cannot be transferred to a contract supplier or any other suppliers.

[43]Capped rental DME items have a limited time period during which they can be rented and paid for by Medicare.

[44]CBP's mail-order diabetic testing supplies and enteral nutrition product categories cannot be grandfathered. CMS announced in December 2011 that Medicare claims submitted for maintenance and servicing of enteral nutrition pumps during 2011 would be paid if the non-contract supplier furnished the pump to a beneficiary in a competitive bidding area and the pump had been rented for at least 15 continuous months at the time of CBP's implementation on January 1, 2011. The supplier that provided the pump in the 15th month of the rental period is responsible for furnishing, maintaining, and servicing the pump—whether it is a contract supplier or not—until the pump is no longer medically necessary for the beneficiary or reaches the end of its reasonable useful lifetime.

Subcontractor Suppliers

Subcontracting allows contract suppliers to work with suppliers that are Medicare-accredited to provide limited services to CBP-covered beneficiaries.[45] A supplier that subcontracts may perform only three services: (1) purchase inventory and fill orders, fabricate or fit items from its own inventory or contract with other companies to purchase items necessary to fill an order, (2) deliver CBP-covered items to beneficiaries, and (3) repair rented equipment. For CBP, subcontracting suppliers may include suppliers that did not bid, that bid and lost, or that won contracts but subcontract with other contract suppliers for a product category not won. The contract suppliers are responsible for billing Medicare for any services that their subcontract suppliers perform since subcontract suppliers are not eligible to bill Medicare themselves. Contract suppliers are to disclose to CMS each subcontracting agreement and are also responsible for ensuring that their subcontractors are Medicare-accredited for the product categories covered by the subcontracting agreement.

Specialty Suppliers

Skilled nursing facilities (SNF)[46] and nursing facilities (NF)[47] are the only entities that can bid to win a CBP contract as a CBP specialty supplier. If such a facility wins a specialty supplier contract, the facility can only furnish the CBP enteral nutrients, equipment, and supplies product category to its own residents covered under Medicare Part B. The facilities may also choose to submit bids to win CBP contracts as a regular contract supplier. If they win a regular contract, they may then furnish the CBP-covered items in the product category they have won to beneficiaries throughout their competitive bidding area.

---

[45]Subcontracting is not limited to CBP; any enrolled DME supplier that bills Medicare for the item it furnishes may subcontract certain services consistent with the DME supplier standards.

[46]A SNF provides residents with restorative services such as physical or speech therapy. A SNF provides a level of care distinguishable from the intensive care furnished by a general hospital or the custodial or supportive care furnished by nursing homes primarily designed to provide daily services above the level of room and board.

[47]A NF provides residents with skilled nursing care and related services for those who require medical or nursing care, rehabilitation of injured, disabled, or sick persons, or on a regular basis, health-related care and services to individuals who because of their mental or physical condition require care and services above the level of room and board. Neither a SNF nor a NF can be a facility that primarily cares for and treats mental diseases.

CBP Online Contract Supplier Locator

To assist beneficiaries in locating a contract supplier in their competitive bidding area, CMS maintains a CBP supplier locator tool on the Medicare website.[48] The supplier locator contains the names of the contract suppliers in each competitive bidding area and the product categories for which they furnish CBP-covered items. The contract suppliers submit information to CMS each quarter on a form that lists the specific items they furnish—including the brand names and equipment models which CMS uses to update the supplier locator.

CBP Beneficiary Assistance through 1-800-MEDICARE

Beneficiaries with CBP questions—referred to by CMS as inquiries—are directed to call 1-800-MEDICARE. Callers are assisted by CBP customer service representatives (CSR) trained to answer questions about CBP in general and to assist beneficiaries in finding CBP suppliers. Beneficiaries calling from area codes in competitive bidding areas hear a prompt at the beginning of their call, which takes them directly to a CBP CSR. Beneficiaries calling from an area code not in a competitive bidding area can also reach a CBP CSR through a series of prompts.

CSRs use CBP scripts—written responses to commonly asked questions—when initially responding to CBP-related calls.[49] CSRs read a response to the beneficiary either from a script about CBP in general, or from a script specific to one of the nine product categories.[50] If the beneficiary's inquiry cannot be addressed by the scripts, the CSR will forward it to an advanced-level CSR trained to research a CBP-related question and respond after completing research on the caller's inquiry. For example, an advanced CSR might work with a beneficiary traveling

---

[48]The tool is located at www.medicare.gov/supplier/.

[49]Scripts address topics that may arise during a beneficiary call to 1-800-MEDICARE regarding CBP, and cover issues such as urgent needs for new supplies, and beneficiaries who are unable to locate a contract supplier in their area. The scripts instruct CSRs how to assist beneficiaries; for example, when a CSR conducts a three-way call with a beneficiary and a contract supplier, the CSR will read a script that says, "My name is [CSR NAME] from 1-800-MEDICARE. I have a beneficiary on the line who is looking for [NAME THE SUPPLY]. His/her name is [BENEFICIARY NAME] and he/she called us because [REASON]. We are calling you because [EXPLAIN THE ISSUE AND WHAT THE SUPPLIER CAN DO TO HELP]."

[50]A single encounter between a caller and a CSR may be counted as more than one inquiry, since an inquiry is counted by the number of scripts which the CSR uses to respond to the call. The number of inquiries does not reflect the number of unique beneficiaries who called.

outside a competitive bidding area to ensure the beneficiary continues to receive necessary DME.

CMS defines a CBP complaint as a CBP inquiry that cannot be resolved by any CSR with 1-800-MEDICARE and is sent to another entity for resolution. The CBP-related entities include: Palmetto GBA, the CMS regional offices, and the CAO.[51] Palmetto GBA investigates all beneficiary or supplier complaints related to alleged CBP contract violations, supplier or quality standard violations, and CBP and Medicare program violations, including fraud and abuse. CMS's regional offices are the focal point for unresolved calls; for example, the offices may assist when a CSR is unable to help a beneficiary find a contract supplier. The CAO responds to other unresolved CBP questions from both suppliers and individuals.

CMS's CBP Monitoring Activities

CMS conducts several monitoring activities to determine whether beneficiary access or satisfaction have been affected by the implementation of CBP. CMS monitors outcomes such as hospitalizations, physician visits, and deaths for beneficiaries in competitive bidding areas, because these outcomes may reflect issues with beneficiary access to necessary DME.[52] CMS posts to its Web site monthly reports on these outcomes in competitive bidding areas and in comparison areas to demonstrate the effects of CBP on health outcomes. CMS also conducted a pre and post-implementation survey to measure beneficiary satisfaction with CBP. The pre-implementation survey was conducted from June 24 to August 3, 2010, and the post-implementation survey was conducted from August 29 to October 20, 2011. CMS surveyed beneficiaries in the nine CBP competitive bidding areas as well as nine comparison markets, chosen to allow a comparison with competitive bidding areas.[53] CMS may also conduct secret shopping in

[51]The CAO program is within the Office of the Medicare Beneficiary Ombudsman, which is responsible for resolving inquiries and complaints for all aspects of the Medicare program.

[52]CMS publicizes health status monitoring results publicly available on its website at http://www.cms.gov/DMEPOSCompetitiveBid/01A3_Monitoring.asp#TopOfPage.

[53]For example, for the Cincinnati competitive bidding area, CMS chose Indianapolis, Indiana as the comparison market.

response to complaints such as those concerning diabetic testing suppliers.[54]

Outcomes of CMS's Implementation of the CBP Round 1 Rebid

The number of bidding suppliers and the number of contracts awarded in the CBP round 1 rebid were very similar to CBP round 1. Improvements were made to the bidding process for the CBP round 1 rebid, and significantly fewer bids were disqualified; nevertheless, many suppliers still had difficulty meeting bid requirements. As in round 1, some suppliers that requested that CMS review their disqualified bids were found to have been incorrectly disqualified and offered a contract.

Nearly the Same Number of Suppliers Bid As in Round 1, and About the Same Percentage of Submitted Bids Resulted in Contracts

Nearly the same number of suppliers bid in both CBP round 1 (1,010 suppliers) and the CBP round 1 rebid (1,011 suppliers). About a third of all the suppliers that bid were awarded at least one CBP contract, and CMS generally met its target—that 30 percent of the suppliers awarded a contract for each product category in each competitive bidding area be small—by awarding contracts to 219 small suppliers of the 356 winning suppliers.[55,56] (See table 1.)

---

[54]In secret shopping, individuals posing as beneficiaries request items such as specific diabetic supplies from contract suppliers to determine whether the suppliers offer the supplies they say they furnish.

[55]To meet CMS's 30 percent target for small supplier participation, small suppliers with bids that originally lost on price could be offered a contract if there were an insufficient number of small suppliers that won on price alone for each product category in each competitive bidding area. CMS's inclusion of small suppliers that originally lost on price did not affect the original single payment amounts.

[56]In CBP round 1, 63 percent of the total number of suppliers that bid and were awarded at least one contract were small.

Table 1: CBP Round 1 Rebid Contract Awards by Supplier Size as of November 3, 2010

Size of bidders	Number of bidders	Percentage of bidders	Number of bidders awarded contracts	Percentage of bidders awarded contracts
Small suppliers	619	61	219	62[a]
Large suppliers	340	34	137	38
Unknown	52	5	0	0
Total	**1,011**	**100**	**356**	**100**

Source: CMS and Palmetto GBA data as of November 3, 2010.

Notes: Categories characterizing size are based on revenue reported on suppliers' financial documents. Small suppliers reported gross revenues of $3.5 million or less in both Medicare and non-Medicare revenues and large suppliers reported more than $3.5 million in both Medicare and non-Medicare revenues. Bidders that did not report this information or submitted bid packages with missing financial documents are categorized as unknown.

[a]According to CMS, 219 small suppliers—or 62 percent of all winning suppliers—received 51 percent of the total 1,217 contracts awarded as of November 3, 2010.

The number of bids that were disqualified in the initial bid review and, therefore, not eligible to compete on price was significantly less in CBP round 1 rebid than in CBP round 1. In CBP round 1 rebid, about 30 percent of bids submitted were disqualified for at least one or more reasons (1,854 of 6,215 submitted). Therefore, about 70 percent of all bids submitted were qualified and used to determine the pivotal bid, which was then used to establish single payment amounts for each item that was included in the CBP round 1 rebid.[57] In contrast, in CBP round 1, almost 50 percent of bids submitted were disqualified during the initial bid review (3,143 of 6,374 submitted) and only about half of all bids submitted were qualified to compete on price.

About 20 percent of bids submitted in the CBP round 1 rebid resulted in contracts between CMS and suppliers (1,217 out of 6,215)—which is comparable to 22 percent of bids that resulted in contracts between CMS and suppliers in CBP round 1 (1,372 out of 6,374.) (See table 2 for round 1 rebid results.)

---

[57]Because the median price of all bids equal or less than the pivotal bid was used to set single payment amounts for all competitively bid items, Medicare's CBP payment amount could be less or more than a particular winning supplier's actual bid for an item.

Table 2: CBP Round 1 Rebid Bid Counts by Process Step as of November 3, 2010

Process step	Number of round 1 rebid bids	Percentage of total bids reviewed
1. Bid review		
Bids reviewed	6,215	100%
Bids disqualified on initial review[a]	(1,854)	29.8
2. Winner selection		
Qualified bids used to determine pivotal bids	4,361	70.2
Bids that lost only on price	(3,074)	49.5
Bids that won on price, were contracts with small suppliers added to meet 30 percent target, or both	1,287	20.7
3. Contract offers		
Initial round of contract offers	1,287	20.7
Contract offers rescinded by CMS after initial round[b]	(11)	0.2
Additional contract offers extended[c]	48	0.8
4. Contract outcomes		
Total contract offers made	1,324	21.3
Contract offers rejected by suppliers[d]	(107)	1.7
Final contracts	1,217	19.6

Source: GAO analysis of CMS data as of November 3, 2010.

Notes: Numbers in parentheses are decreases. The number of bids submitted is higher than the number of bidding suppliers because suppliers could submit bids in multiple product categories and multiple competitive bidding areas.

[a]Some of the bids that were disqualified during the initial bid review would have lost on price had they not been disqualified for at least one other reason. Some bids that were disqualified during the initial bid review were later found to have been incorrectly disqualified.

[b]CMS made these contract offers, but later rescinded them because CMS found that commonly-controlled or owned suppliers had submitted separate bids for the same product category in the same competitive bidding area. These suppliers were disqualified because suppliers are prohibited by CMS from bidding against themselves for the same product category in the same competitive bidding area.

[c]After 107 contract offers were rejected, CMS extended additional contract offers to small suppliers in specific product categories and competitive bidding areas to meet CMS's 30 percent target for small supplier participation.

[d]CMS extended these contract offers, but suppliers did not accept them.

CMS made initial contract offers for CBP round 1 rebid within the 3-month period between July 1, 2010, and September 24, 2010, and announced the winning contract suppliers on November 3, 2010. Although CBP round 1 rebid contracts began on January 1, 2011, CMS made additional contract offers between December 17, 2010, and January 24, 2011.

Despite Improvements and Fewer Bid Disqualifications, Many Suppliers Still Had Difficulty Meeting Bid Requirements

Fewer bids were disqualified in CBP round 1 rebid and CMS provided additional feedback to suppliers that had bids disqualified, indicating to suppliers all the reasons for disqualification. While CMS improved the CBP bidding process, many suppliers still had difficulty complying with bid submission requirements, and had particular difficulty with financial documentation requirements. Although the majority of suppliers with disqualified bids that contacted CMS with questions were found to have been correctly disqualified, some suppliers were later found to have incorrectly disqualified bids and were offered contracts.

Fewer Bids Were Disqualified in CBP Round 1 Rebid

About 20 percent fewer bids were disqualified during the initial bid review of CBP round 1 rebid than in round 1. The number of bids disqualified in CBP round 1 rebid would have been higher if many suppliers had not benefited from a new process giving suppliers the opportunity to be notified of and submit missing required financial documentation[58]—a process that was not available during CBP round 1.

Suppliers had bids disqualified for one or more reasons, and for the CBP round 1 rebid CMS increased its feedback to suppliers by using 11 general reason codes—four more than were used in CBP round 1—to provide feedback to suppliers that had bids disqualified. For example, 109 distinct[59] suppliers had 356 bids disqualified because they did not meet all state licensure requirements in every state of the competitive bidding areas for the product category in which they submitted bids. (See table 3.) In November 2010, CMS sent a letter to suppliers that were not offered a CBP contract notifying them of all the reasons that their bids were disqualified, including whether their bids would have lost on price—

[58]Financial documentation means a financial, tax, or other document required to be submitted in order to meet CMS's financial standards for CBP.

[59]The term distinct is used to indicate a supplier that is not being double-counted. For example, if a supplier had multiple bids disqualified because the bids did not meet licensure requirements, the supplier is only counted one time for having bids disqualified for that reason. If a supplier had a bid disqualified for two or more reasons, the supplier would be counted as one distinct supplier for each reason that its bids were disqualified.

either for that reason alone or in addition to another bid submission deficiency reason.[60]

Table 3: Number and Percentage of CBP Round 1 Rebid Disqualified Bids by Reason for Disqualification as of November 3, 2010

Reason for bid disqualification	Bids disqualified during initial bid review	Percentage of bids disqualified[a]
Unacceptable (incomplete or inaccurate) financial documentation (Suppliers failed to submit hardcopy financial documentation as required)	834	45%
Did not meet all state licensure requirements (Suppliers were responsible for meeting all applicable state licensure requirements for the product category in every state of a competitive bidding areas they submitted a bid)	356	19
Did not meet supplier financial standards (Supplier financial standards indicated that CMS believed that the supplier was unlikely for financial reasons to be able to fulfill its contract obligations)	293	16
Missing required hardcopy documentation (Suppliers must submit financial documentation in hardcopy)	216	12
Bid price for one or more item was deemed not bona fide (All bid prices could not be higher than the Medicare fee schedule but not lower than the cost to the supplier)	169	9
Did not meet accreditation requirements (Suppliers must have been accredited by a CMS-approved accreditation organization for the product categories in which they submitted bids)	71	4
National Supplier Clearinghouse (NSC) number was revoked or inactive (Suppliers must have had an active NSC number to be eligible to bill Medicare for DME)	65	4
Did not meet common ownership rules[b] (Commonly-owned or controlled suppliers were required to submit a single bid to furnish a product category in a competitive bidding area)	16	<1
Did not meet network criteria (A network is a group of between two to 20 small suppliers that collectively submit a bid as a single entity and must meet certain criteria—including that they cannot independently furnish all of the items in the product category for which the network is submitting a bid to beneficiaries throughout the entire geographic area of the competitive bidding area)	12	<1

[60]A CMS official told us CMS changed the way it reported bid disqualifications for CBP round 1 rebid by establishing a CBP bid disqualification hierarchy that ranks a supplier's bid disqualifications on the basis of the reason codes. Although a supplier that had a bid disqualified for more than one reason was notified of all reasons, the CMS official told us that CMS only counted a bid that was disqualified for more than one reason code once—under the highest reason code of the hierarchy. If a bid was disqualified for any reason, but would have also lost on price, CMS included it under the "lost on price" reason code—the highest code of its hierarchy.

Reason for bid disqualification	Bids disqualified during initial bid review	Percentage of bids disqualified[a]
Did not meet eligibility requirements to bid as a specialty supplier (A specialty supplier is a skilled nursing facility or nursing facility that is awarded a competitive bidding contract to furnish competitively bid items only to its own residents to whom it would otherwise furnish Medicare Part B services)	0	0

Source: GAO analysis of CMS data as of November 3, 2010.

Notes: CMS issued CBP round 1 rebid bid instructions to inform suppliers about bid submission requirements.

In addition to the reasons for bid disqualification above, CMS also established a "lost on price" category. According to CMS, 1,273 of the 1,854 total bids disqualified—69 percent—would also have lost on price had the bid not been disqualified for at least one other reason.

[a]Percentages add to more than 100 because a bid could be disqualified for more than one reason.

[b]Two or more suppliers are commonly-owned if one or more of them has an ownership interest totaling at least five percent of the other supplier. A supplier controls another supplier if one or more of its owners is an officer, director, or partner in the other.

Despite Improvements, Many Suppliers Had Difficulty with Financial Documentation Requirements

Although fewer bids were disqualified in CBP round 1 rebid, many suppliers had difficulty meeting the bidding requirements. As occurred in CBP round 1, in which 88 percent of disqualified bids were disqualified because they failed to provide the required financial documentation or did not meet CMS's minimum financial standard threshold for suppliers, the majority of CBP round 1 rebid bids (73 percent) that were disqualified on initial bid review were also disqualified for the same reasons.[61]

Specifically, 44 distinct suppliers (about 4 percent of all bidding suppliers) had 293 bids disqualified because the bidding suppliers did not meet CMS's minimum supplier financial standards. Bidding suppliers that did not meet minimum financial standards would be unlikely for financial reasons to be able to fulfill their contract obligations, in CMS's judgment. In addition, 162 distinct suppliers (about 16 percent of all bidding suppliers) submitted 834 bids that were disqualified because of unacceptable or inaccurate financial documentation, while 51 distinct suppliers (about 5 percent of all bidding suppliers) submitted 216 bids with missing financial documentation.

The number of CBP round 1 rebid bids disqualified for missing financial documentation would have been higher without CMS's implementation of the MIPPA provision for financial document review. Under this provision,

---

[61]These bids may also have been disqualified for one or more other reasons.

CMS is required to determine if any suppliers' financial documents that are submitted by a certain time in a CBP bid window—known as the covered document review date[62]—are missing and to notify and provide suppliers the opportunity to submit them.[63] In CBP round 1 rebid, 791 suppliers—or 78 percent of all bidding suppliers—submitted their financial documentation by the covered document review date. Of those eligible to have their financial documentation reviewed, 321 suppliers (about 41 percent) were notified that they had missing documentation—including 184 small suppliers. Of the 321 suppliers that were notified, 232 suppliers submitted the correct missing documentation, 14 did not provide missing documentation, and 75 resubmitted their documentation, but were ultimately disqualified for unacceptable (such as incomplete or inaccurate) documents. Ninety-three of the 321 suppliers—about 29 percent—that were notified by CMS that they had missing financial documentation, and subsequently provided correct documentation, were ultimately awarded one or more CBP contracts.

In both CBP round 1 and the CBP round 1 rebid, the statement of cash flow[64] was the most common reason that suppliers were disqualified for missing or unacceptable financial documentation. Although CMS provided an example of a statement of cash flow in the CBP round 1 rebid bidding instructions and suggested that financial statements be compiled by an independent accounting firm or prepared by the supplier, Palmetto GBA reported that it was obvious that many bidding suppliers still did not understand what constituted an acceptable statement of cash flow during the CBP round 1 rebid bid submission process. According to CMS, one reason that the statement of cash flow was the most difficult financial

---

[62]MIPPA and implementing regulations define the covered document review date as the later of: (1) 30 days before the final date for the close of the bid window; or (2) 30 days after the bid window opens. For CBP round 1 rebid, CMS was required to notify eligible suppliers of missing financial documentation within 45 days after the end of the covered document review date. For future rounds, CMS must notify eligible suppliers of missing financial documentation within 90 days after the end of the covered document review date. MIPPA provided that the covered document review date only applies to the timely submission of financial documentation and does not apply to any determination by CMS as to the accuracy or completeness of the documentation submitted or whether the documents meet applicable financial requirements.

[63]Once notified, suppliers have 10 business days to submit missing financial documentation.

[64]The statement of cash flow contains 1 year of information for operating, financing, and investing activities and the beginning and ending cash balances.

document to prepare in both CBP rounds is because it is prepared much less often than other types of financial documents—particularly by small suppliers. CMS reported that another obstacle in preparing acceptable statements of cash flow is that suppliers with very limited understanding of accounting practices and how to prepare financial statements compiled the statements of cash flow themselves and relied on results generated by inexpensive accounting software, which CMS told us was not sufficient. As a result, CMS provided additional information in its CBP round 2 bidding instructions, and strongly recommended that suppliers' financial statements be compiled by an independent accounting firm to discourage suppliers from preparing their own financial documents.

As in Round 1, CMS Found through Its Clarified Postbidding Review Process That Some Suppliers' Round 1 Rebid Bids Were Incorrectly Disqualified

In the CBP round 1 rebid, as in CBP round 1, CMS determined that some suppliers' bids had been incorrectly disqualified. During CBP round 1, we reported that CMS did not effectively communicate to suppliers that they had an opportunity to have their round 1 bids reviewed. CMS officials told us that they conducted a postbidding review process for suppliers which contacted the agency with questions or requested a review and subsequently found that 10 of the 357 round 1 suppliers that had bids reviewed had been incorrectly disqualified. After reviewing the language that CMS provided to suppliers during CBP round 1, we determined that CMS did not effectively communicate to suppliers that they had an opportunity to have disqualified round 1 bids reviewed. As a result, in 2009, we recommended, and CMS agreed, that if CMS chose to conduct a review of disqualification decisions during CBP round 1 rebid and future bids, CMS should notify and give all suppliers an equal opportunity for review, and clearly indicate how suppliers can request a review.[65]

---

[65]Specifically, we recommended that to improve future rounds of the CBP, and if CMS decided to conduct a review of disqualification decisions during the CBP round 1 rebid and future rounds, CMS should notify all suppliers of any such process, give suppliers equal opportunity for such reviews, and clearly indicate how they can request a review. CMS responded that it agreed that all suppliers should receive notice about all aspects of the CBP and noted that all CBP round 1 bidders were specifically advised in writing of the opportunity to ask questions about their bid results. CMS also stated that it continues to believe that suppliers should have the opportunity to raise questions or concerns about the CBP, including disqualification decisions. Further, CMS stated that it continues to believe that the competitive bidding statute and regulations permit CMS to conduct quality assurance checks during the course of responding to bidders' questions as part of CMS's other extensive quality assurance efforts and that CMS remained committed to answering suppliers' questions and will continue to ensure that all suppliers are sufficiently informed about opportunities for the CBP round 1 rebid and future rounds. See GAO-10-27.

Although the notification that CMS provided to suppliers during the CBP round 1 rebid provided more information than was provided during CBP round 1, CMS did not inform suppliers that a review of a disqualified bid could possibly result in reversal of the disqualification and extension of a contract offer. (See fig. 2.)

Figure 2: Excerpts from the Letters CMS Sent Bidding Suppliers Regarding the Opportunity for Postbid Review of Disqualified Bids in CBP Round 1 and CBP Round 1 Rebid

CBP round 1:

If you have any questions, please contact the customer service center at 877-577-5331.[a]

CBP round 1 rebid:

CMS believes that suppliers should have the opportunity to raise questions or concerns about the competitive bidding process, including disqualification decisions. Therefore, we are providing a targeted period for suppliers to ask questions or express concerns about the reasons(s) why they were not awarded a contract. If you have any questions or concerns regarding your bid(s), please contact the customer service center at 877-577-5331 by November 19, 2010.[b]

Source: CMS.

[a]In CBP round 1, CMS sent a separate letter to suppliers that lost on price and suppliers that had bids disqualified for at least one other reason.

[b]In the CBP round 1 rebid, CMS sent the same letter to suppliers that lost on price and had disqualified bids, and indicated all the reasons a supplier's bid was disqualified—including whether the bid would have lost on price. CMS announced winning suppliers on November 3, 2010, so suppliers were given about 2 weeks to call the customer service center with questions or concerns regarding their losing bids. However, Palmetto GBA reported that it was continuing to receive inquiries from suppliers that had bids disqualified in CBP round 1 rebid as of June 17, 2011.

In both CBP rounds, CMS determined that some suppliers that contacted Palmetto GBA and requested a review of their bids had been incorrectly disqualified. (See table 4.) CMS told us it received bid inquiries from 99 suppliers that had bids disqualified in CBP round 1 rebid and subsequently extended contracts to 7 of those suppliers—about 7 percent. In CBP round 1, 10 suppliers—or 3 percent of the 357 suppliers that contacted Palmetto GBA—were found to have bids that were incorrectly disqualified.[66] Suppliers' bids could have been incorrectly disqualified for various reasons, such as for issues regarding financial documentation, because they were thought not to have the required license in the state or product category in which bids were submitted, or because the bids were deemed not bona fide.[67]

Table 4: Results of CMS's Post-Bid Review Process in CBP Round 1 and CBP Round 1 Rebid

Postbid review	CBP round 1	CBP round 1 rebid
Total number of bids submitted	6,374	6,215
Total number of bidding suppliers	1,010	1,011
Total number of suppliers that requested a review	357	99[a]
Total number of suppliers that were found to have bids that were incorrectly disqualified	10[b]	7
Percentage of suppliers that were offered a contract as a result of the post-bid review	3%	7%

Source: GAO analysis of CMS and Palmetto GBA data.

[a]Palmetto GBA reported that the decrease in the number of disqualified suppliers that requested a post-bid review during CBP round 1 rebid can be partly attributed to CMS indicating which disqualified bids would have lost on price if not disqualified for at least one other reason.

[b]Ten suppliers were found to have been incorrectly disqualified, and 7 suppliers were offered contracts because they had bids equal to or less than the pivotal bid or were needed to meet CMS's target for small supplier participation.

Effects on Suppliers of the First Year of the CBP Round 1 Rebid

Both contract and non-contract suppliers have been affected by the first year of the CBP round 1 rebid. In the first months of 2011, few CBP contract suppliers had their contracts terminated by CMS, voluntarily canceled their contracts, or were involved in ownership changes. Since the CBP round 1 rebid began, many non-contract suppliers have chosen

---

[66]Of the 10 suppliers that were incorrectly disqualified in CBP round 1, 7 suppliers were offered contracts for 27 bids because they had bids equal to or less than the pivotal bid or were needed to meet CMS's small supplier participation goal.

[67]All bids must be bona fide, meaning that they cannot be higher than the Medicare fee schedule or lower than the supplier's cost.

to be grandfathered suppliers for certain CBP rental DME. Some contract and non-contract suppliers have entered into subcontracting agreements to provide certain services to beneficiaries in CBP competitive bidding areas. Some suppliers with no previous experience with the DME product category or no location in a competitive bidding area were awarded contracts as CBP allows.

Four Percent of the Original Contract Suppliers Had Contracts Terminated or Canceled in CBP's First 10 Months of 2011

During the first 10 months of 2011, 16 of the original 356 contract suppliers—4 percent—left CBP due to CMS terminating contract suppliers (8), or from contract suppliers voluntarily canceling their CBP contracts (8). (See table 5.) The 16 contract suppliers had 28 affected CBP contracts—about 2 percent of the 1,217 original CBP contracts. Thirteen of the 16 contract suppliers were small suppliers.

Table 5: CBP Round 1 Rebid Contract Supplier Terminations and Cancelations, January 1 through October 31, 2011

Termination and cancelation reasons	Number of CBP contract suppliers	Number of CBP contracts
CMS terminations		
• National Supplier Clearinghouse (NSC)[a] revoked supplier's PTAN (provider transaction access number)	3	5
• Contract supplier non-operational and not accredited	1	5
• Contract supplier losing accreditation	2	3
• Contract supplier being inactivated or non-operational	2	3
Contract supplier cancelations[b]		
• Contract supplier being inactive and voluntarily withdrew from Medicare	7	8
• Contract supplier had a change of ownership and voluntarily withdrew from Medicare	1	4
Total	**16**	**28**

Source: GAO analysis of CMS data.

[a]The NSC is a CMS contractor responsible for DMEPOS supplier enrollment in Medicare and may revoke a supplier's enrollment, for example, if a supplier loses its Medicare accreditation.

[b]Effective July 1, 2011, CMS decided to report contracts as canceled rather than terminated when the contract supplier voluntarily withdrew from Medicare through the NSC.

CBP contracts can be terminated by CMS when a contract supplier fails to meet CBP requirements, for example, when Medicare accreditation is not maintained. A contract supplier can end its CBP contracts by voluntarily withdrawing from Medicare. For example, one contract supplier testified at a CMS CBP Program Advisory and Oversight Committee (PAOC) meeting that it had bid on numerous product categories but won only one contract and would be closing its business due to lost revenue; the supplier withdrew from Medicare in May 2011.

Twenty-one of the 28 contracts involved two competitive bidding areas—Miami (15) and Riverside (6). Eighteen contracts involved two product categories—oxygen (10) and standard power wheelchairs (8). The Riverside competitive bidding area had six of the eight standard power wheelchair contracts that were ended.

Eight DME Contract Supplier Ownership Changes Occurred in CBP's First 11 Months

Eight DME supplier ownership changes—about 2 percent of the original 356 contract suppliers—occurred from November 3, 2010, when the winning contract suppliers were first announced, through November 30, 2011.[68] While contract suppliers can be sold, their CBP contracts cannot. If a contract supplier's ownership changes, CMS decides whether the CBP contract can be assumed by the new purchasing supplier—which can be another contract supplier or a non-contract supplier—by determining if the purchasing supplier meets the CBP contract supplier standards. In all nine changes, CMS determined that the new owners would assume the CBP contracts involved. (See table 6.)

Table 6: Eight Ownership Changes Involving CBP Contract Suppliers, November 3, 2010, through November 3, 2011

Supplier ownership change transaction	Which supplier assumes the involved CBP contract	Total
Non-contract supplier purchases a contract supplier	CMS allows the purchasing non-contract supplier to assume the purchased contract supplier's contract or contracts	4
Contract supplier purchases another contract supplier	CMS allows the purchasing contract supplier to assume the purchased contract supplier's contract or contracts	4

Source: GAO analysis of CMS data.

[68]A change in ownership results in either (a) a new entity or company that did not exist before the merger or acquisition transaction; or (b) a successor entity or company that exists before the transaction, merges or acquires a contract supplier, and continues to exist as it did before the transaction. For this discussion, we use the terms purchase or bought to include both acquisitions and mergers.

GAO-12-693 DME Competitive Bidding Program

CBP Grandfathering Option Temporarily Affects Medicare Revenues for Some Suppliers

The CBP provides a grandfathering option that temporarily benefits some non-contract suppliers while also temporarily disadvantaging some contract suppliers. For non-contract suppliers, grandfathering allows them to retain Medicare revenues for some CBP-covered capped rental DME items for the length of the items' rental periods, if the beneficiary involved chooses to remain with the grandfathered supplier until the rental period expires. For contract suppliers that won CBP contracts for the same DME capped rental DME items, grandfathering may be a temporary disadvantage in both limiting the number of Medicare beneficiaries they can serve and the amount of Medicare revenue they can immediately try to gain. Unless the beneficiary served by a grandfathered supplier decides to choose a contract supplier, the contract suppliers cannot try to furnish items to the same beneficiary and thus cannot increase their CBP Medicare revenue as quickly as they may have anticipated.

The degree of grandfathering varies among the allowed product categories and competitive bidding areas.[69] In CBP's first 11 months of 2011, the top three grandfathered product categories—both by the number of beneficiaries renting items and by the allowed Medicare payments to grandfathered suppliers—were CPAP/RAD,[70] hospital beds, and oxygen.[71] (See table 7.)

---

[69]CMS determines the grandfathered suppliers by whether they are submitting Medicare claims for furnishing CBP-covered DME items to the same beneficiary they were before CBP began on January 1, 2011.

[70]CPAP/RAD means continuous positive airway pressure devices and respiratory assist devices; CPAP may be used, for example, to treat sleep apnea.

[71]Since oxygen is rented for a much longer time period than the 13-month capped rental period, CMS decided grandfathered suppliers for oxygen would be paid at CBP single payment amounts; grandfathering suppliers furnishing capped rental items and inexpensive and routinely purchased DME are paid at the Medicare fee schedule.

Table 7: Top Three Grandfathered Product Categories, CBP Round 1 Rebid, January 2011 and November 2011 Compared

Product category (rental items only)	Beneficiaries continuing to rent from the same supplier as before CBP		Allowed Medicare payments to grandfathered non-contract suppliers	
	January	November	January	November
Oxygen	16,732	4,952	$2,167,352	$627,069
Hospital beds	9,462	850	976,108	81,289
CPAP/RAD	8,558	1,294	903,996	105,791
Total	**34,752**	**7,096**	**$4,047,456**	**$814,149**

Source: GAO analysis of CMS and CMS's Pricing, Data Analysis and Coding contractor data as of November 30, 2011.

The number of grandfathered suppliers has generally steadily declined during 2011 as rental periods expire or beneficiaries chose contract suppliers. In January 2011 when the CBP round 1 rebid began, there were 1,364 grandfathered suppliers or 58 percent of the 2,363 suppliers that billed for beneficiaries they had been serving as of December 31, 2010. In comparison, in December 2011, there were 575 grandfathering suppliers or 22 percent of the 2,594 suppliers that billed for beneficiaries they had been serving as of December 31, 2010. (See fig. 3.)

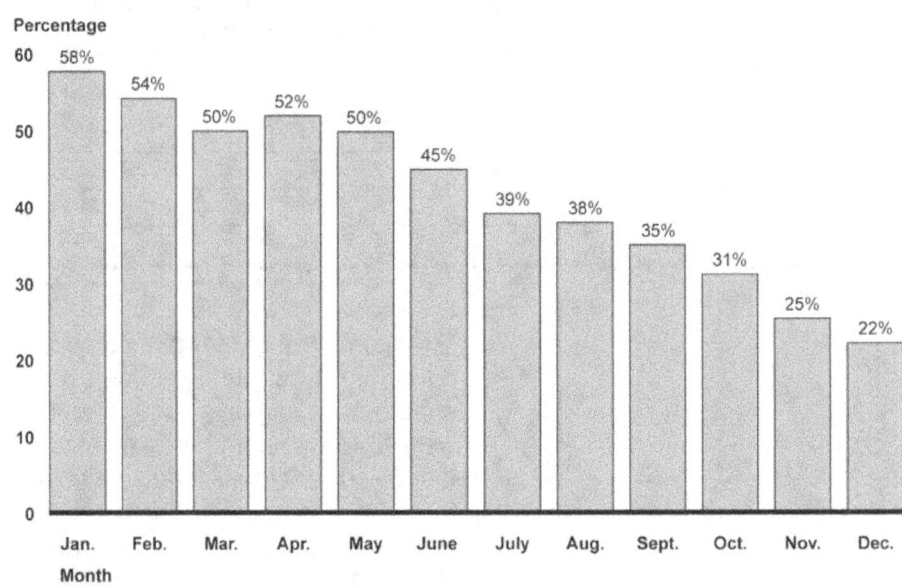

Figure 3: Percentage of DME Suppliers that Grandfathered in CBP Round 1 Rebid by Month, 2011

Source: GAO analysis of data from CMS and CMS's Pricing, Data Analysis and Coding contractor.

Notes: There were 2,363 DME suppliers that submitted Medicare claims in December 2010 for CBP-covered items in the nine CBP competitive bidding areas before CBP began on January 1, 2011. The percentage figure entry for each month is calculated using the number of grandfathering suppliers that submitted eligible Medicare claims that month. The 2011 monthly numbers of grandfathering suppliers fluctuate each month based on when suppliers submitted their Medicare claims.

About 31 Percent of CBP Contract Suppliers Reported They Had Subcontracts with Other Suppliers in CBP's First 8 Months

At the end of July 2011, about 31 percent of contract suppliers had subcontracting agreements. There were 112 distinct[72] contract suppliers that had at least one subcontracting agreement with one of 211 distinct subcontractor suppliers. Four contract suppliers had terminated some of their subcontracts, and three contract suppliers had subcontracting agreements pending CMS approval.

Some contract suppliers that were new to the competitive bidding area where they won or were new to a product category they won have subcontracting agreements with non-contract suppliers. Among the

---

[72]The term distinct is used to indicate that a supplier is not being double-counted. For example, if the same contract supplier has numerous subcontractors, it is counted as one distinct contract supplier that is subcontracting.

44 distinct contract suppliers that did not have a previous business location in the competitive bidding area where they won at least one contract, 30 percent (13 suppliers) had at least one subcontracting agreement with a non-contract supplier. For the 43 distinct contract suppliers that were new to a product category, 37 percent (16 suppliers) had at least one subcontracting agreement.[73]

Although CMS requires contract suppliers to notify it of their subcontracting agreements, contract suppliers do not have to provide CMS with copies of their subcontracting agreements or report what they pay their subcontract suppliers. Contract suppliers are free to negotiate their own subcontracting agreements as CMS does not have subcontracting guidelines or an agreement template. For example, one subcontract supplier told us it negotiated with a contract supplier for a flat rate for hospital bed deliveries of $60 and another subcontract supplier had a $75 rate; one also negotiated a $20 delivery fee for walkers. Two subcontract suppliers told us that they have a 30-day termination notice provision in their agreements with contract suppliers.

As CBP Allows, Some Suppliers with No Previous Experience in a Product Category or with No Location in a Competitive Bidding Area Were Awarded Contracts

As allowed under CBP, CMS awarded round 1 rebid contracts to some suppliers that at the time they bid had no previous experience in at least one product category, or were new to at least one competitive bidding area—did not have a prior business location in the area—or both.[74] There were 43 distinct[75] contract suppliers new to a product category and 44 new to a competitive bidding area—each were about 12 percent of the 356 original contract suppliers awarded contracts. Nine distinct contract suppliers were new to both a product category and a competitive bidding area; four of these were small suppliers.

[73]Although these contract suppliers have subcontracts, it is not known whether the subcontracts are related to the contract supplier not having had prior experience in a product category or not having had a prior business location in the competitive bidding area.

[74]All suppliers offered a CBP contract must be accredited and licensed.

[75]We determined the number of distinct suppliers, since contract suppliers can be counted more than once if they are new to more than one product category or more than one competitive bidding area.

Of the 43 distinct contract suppliers with no previous experience for a product category they won, 23 are small suppliers. The enteral nutrition[76] product category had the most contract suppliers new to a product category—19; the complex power wheelchairs product category had none. (See table 8.)

Table 8: Contract Suppliers New to a Product Category, CBP Round 1 Rebid

	Product category	Contract suppliers new to the product category	Percentage of contract suppliers new to the product category compared to all contract suppliers in the product category
1	Enteral nutrients	19	13%
2	Oxygen and oxygen equipment	10	5
3	Walkers	10	8
4	Hospital beds	9	9
5	CPAP/RAD	6	6
6	Mail-order diabetic supplies	6	29
7	Standard power wheelchairs	5	4
8	Support surfaces (Miami only)	3	21
9	Complex power wheelchairs	0	0
	Total	**68**	

Source: GAO analysis of CMS data.

Notes: Since contract suppliers may be new to more than one product category, some suppliers are counted more than once. Among the 68 contract suppliers new to a product category, there are 43 distinct contract suppliers among the nine product categories. The entries in the percentage column are based on the percentage of contract suppliers that are new to the product category as compared to all contract suppliers in the same product category; the percentage column's entries do not, therefore, add up to 100 percent.

Additionally, 44 distinct contract suppliers were new to a competitive bidding area where they won at least one contract; 18 were small suppliers. While all of the competitive bidding areas had suppliers new to the area, the Cleveland competitive bidding area had the most (21), and the Miami area had the least (3). (See table 9.)

---

[76]Enteral nutrition equipment and supplies are used to provide enteral nutrients through a tube into the stomach or small intestine commonly referred to as tube feeding.

Table 9: Contract Suppliers New to a Competitive Bidding Area, CBP Round 1 Rebid

	Competitive bidding area	Distinct contract suppliers new to the competitive bidding area	Percentage of distinct contract suppliers new to the competitive bidding area compared to all distinct contract suppliers for the area
1	Cleveland	21	34%
2	Pittsburgh	16	26
3	Cincinnati	13	20
4	Charlotte	11	19
5	Kansas City	11	21
6	Orlando	10	15
7	Riverside	8	12
8	Dallas	4	5
9	Miami	3	3
	Total	**97**	

Source: GAO analysis of CMS data.

Notes: Since contract suppliers may be new to more than one competitive bidding area, some suppliers are counted more than once. Among the nine competitive bidding areas, there are 97 suppliers new to areas—44 are distinct contract suppliers. The entries in the percentage column are based on the percentage of contract suppliers that are new to a competitive bidding area as compared to all contract suppliers in the same competitive bidding area; the percentage column's entries do not, therefore, add up to 100 percent.

Although CMS's Monitoring Activities Have Limitations, They Indicate that Beneficiary Access and Satisfaction Have Not Been Affected by CBP

CMS's monitoring efforts reported declining inquiries and complaints over the first year of CBP implementation, high levels of beneficiary satisfaction, and no changes in health outcomes. Although some of these efforts have limitations, in the aggregate, they provide useful information to CMS regarding beneficiary access and satisfaction.

CBP Inquiries and Complaints Decreased During CBP's First Year 2011

Information collected from CMS's monitoring of inquiries to 1-800-MEDICARE suggests that CBP has not adversely affected beneficiary access to or satisfaction with DME. Calls to 1-800-MEDICARE regarding CBP declined during the first year of CBP implementation, and 2 percent of calls were from beneficiaries with an urgent need for CBP-covered DME. CBP-related calls comprised a small fraction of all calls to 1-800-MEDICARE.

In 2011, CMS classified 127,466 CBP-related calls to 1-800-MEDICARE as inquiries. (See fig. 4.) The total number of CBP-related inquiries to 1-800-MEDICARE declined from 19,887 in January 2011 to 4,501 in December 2011. In the first 3 months of CBP implementation, most inquiries were regarding CBP in general. In subsequent months, there were more inquiries about specific CBP-covered products than about CBP generally. Over 2 million beneficiaries were involved in CBP round 1 rebid; the ratio of inquiries to 1-800-MEDICARE compared with CBP beneficiaries is approximately 1 inquiry for every 16 beneficiaries.[77]

---

[77]According to CMS, each beneficiary may make more than one call to 1-800-MEDICARE, and each call would be classified as at least one inquiry. The ratio does not represent the percentage of beneficiaries who called 1-800-MEDICARE.

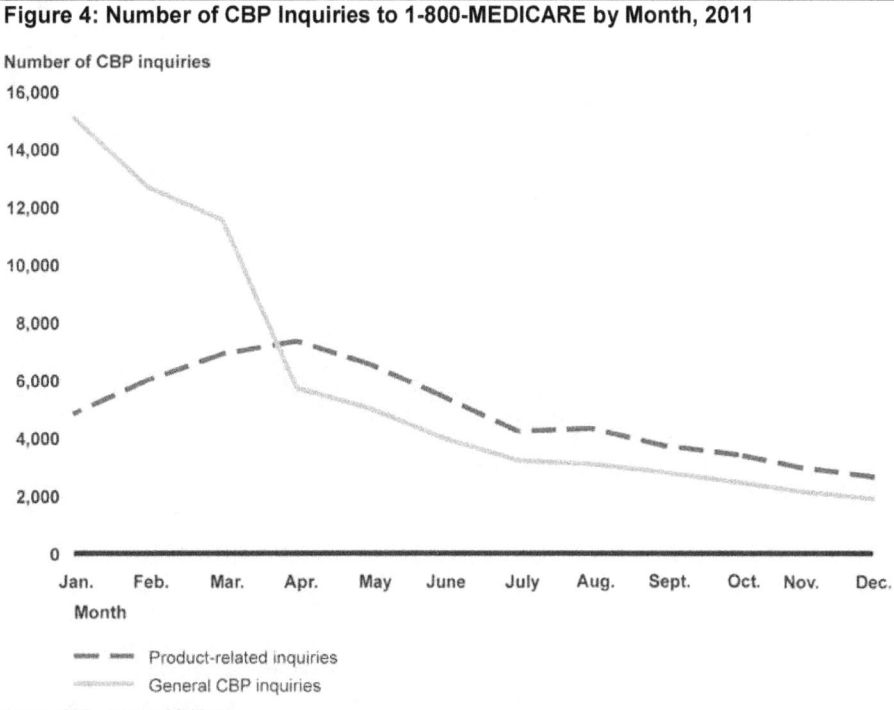

Figure 4: Number of CBP Inquiries to 1-800-MEDICARE by Month, 2011

Number of CBP inquiries

- - - Product-related inquiries
      General CBP inquiries

Source: GAO analysis of CMS data.

Inquiries to 1-800-MEDICARE regarding CBP comprise less than one-half of 1 percent of inquiries to 1-800-MEDICARE. On average, CBP-related calls to 1-800-MEDICARE comprise nearly 13 percent of all DMEPOS-related calls. The proportion of DME-related 1-800-MEDICARE inquiries pertaining to CBP fell in 2011 from 19 percent in the first quarter to less than 7 percent in the fourth quarter. (See fig. 5.) Inquiries and complaints to 1-800-MEDICARE regarding DMEPOS in general, including CBP-related calls, have remained fairly steady from 2010 to 2011.

Figure 5: Percent of CBP-related Inquiries to 1-800-MEDICARE Compared to All DMEPOS-related Inquiries by Quarter, 2011

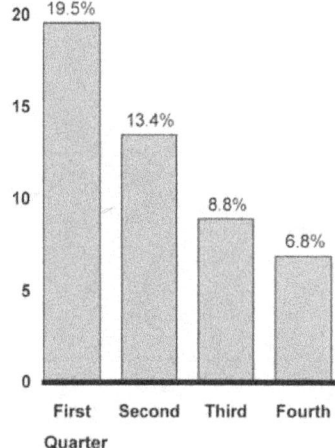

Percentage

Source: GAO analysis of CMS data.

Note: DMEPOS-related inquiries include CBP inquiries.

The majority of product-specific inquiries to 1-800-MEDICARE—over 40,000—were about mail-order diabetic supplies. There were approximately 5,000 inquiries regarding standard power wheelchairs, 4,000 inquiries regarding CPAP/RAD, and 3,000 regarding walkers. (See fig. 6.)

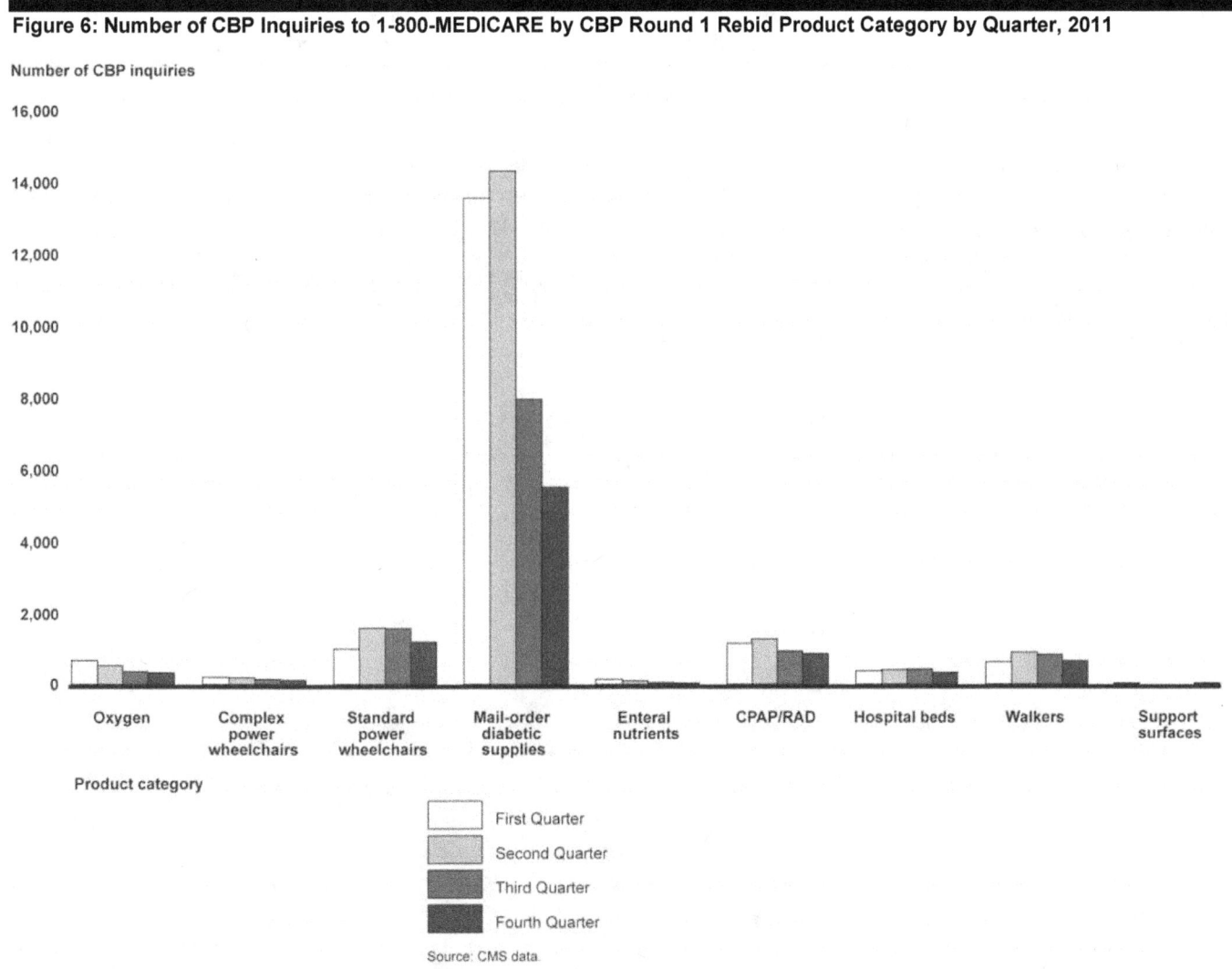

Figure 6: Number of CBP Inquiries to 1-800-MEDICARE by CBP Round 1 Rebid Product Category by Quarter, 2011

Number of CBP inquiries

First Quarter
Second Quarter
Third Quarter
Fourth Quarter

Source: CMS data.

CSRs at 1-800-MEDICARE may respond to beneficiaries with time-sensitive inquiries. In 2011, there were no life-threatening inquiries related to CBP[78] and 2,539 immediate-needs inquiries—about 2 percent of all inquiries. Immediate needs inquiries are defined as situations in which

[78]Life-threatening inquiries are defined as situations in which without assistance, beneficiaries would be unable to access equipment needed immediately to sustain life. In life-threatening situations, CSRs instruct beneficiaries to call 911.

GAO-12-693 DME Competitive Bidding Program

beneficiaries have less than 2 days of life-sustaining DME, or in which beneficiaries' medical condition will be worsened if they are unable to access DME.

CBP Complaints Decreased During 2011, But CMS's Definition of Complaint May Not Reveal Beneficiary Access Problems

In the first year of CBP, CMS classified 151 calls as complaints. (See fig. 7.) Seventy-seven percent of these complaints—or 116 complaints—occurred in the first half of 2011.

Figure 7: CBP Complaints to 1-800-MEDICARE by Quarter, 2011

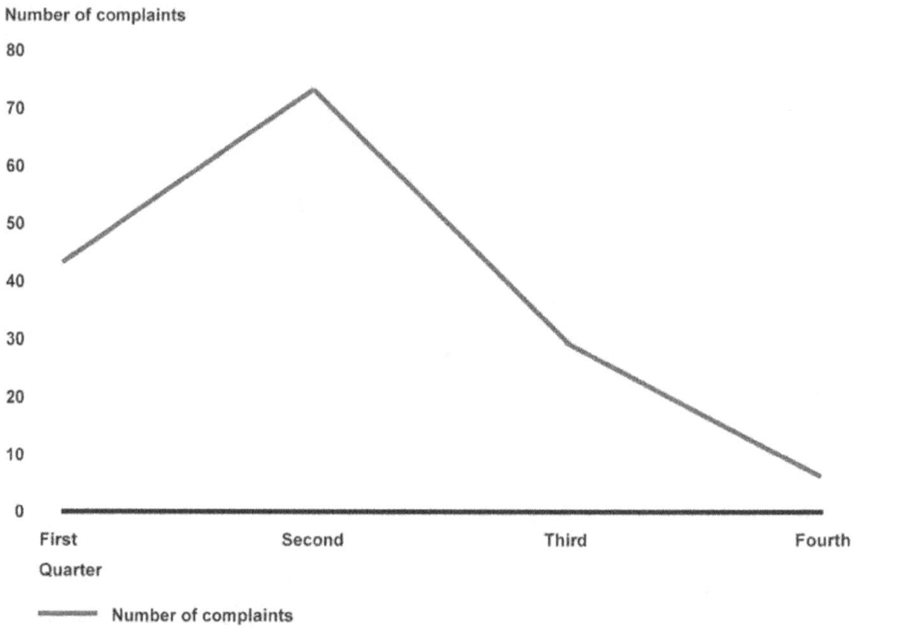

Number of complaints

Source: GAO analysis of CMS data.

CMS's definition of inquiry and complaint may be an optimistic characterization of beneficiary calls. According to CMS, all calls are first classified as inquiries and are only classified as complaints when they remain unresolved by CSRs. However, CSRs are able to address most beneficiary inquiries, so the definition of inquiry encompasses the majority of types of calls to 1-800-MEDICARE. Inquiries may be recorded as complaints because of their level of complexity, rather than as a reflection of beneficiary dissatisfaction. CMS officials told us CSRs may forward complex inquiries to another entity for response, and these inquiries would be classified as complaints regardless of whether the beneficiary intended to log a complaint.

CMS Monitored Beneficiary Satisfaction and Health Outcomes During the First Year of Implementation

CMS has multiple ongoing monitoring efforts to ensure that CBP beneficiaries can access DME and are satisfied with the program. While these tools have limitations, CMS's monitoring of the first year of CBP implementation does not show evidence that beneficiaries have been affected negatively by CBP. Some of these tools—such as the beneficiary satisfaction survey—finished collecting data at the end of 2011. CMS's claims and health outcomes monitoring tool found no changes in health outcomes in competitive bidding areas in 2011, but this method may not fully capture the relationship between access to DME and health outcomes. Other tools—such as secret shopping—are limited in scope, so their data will not provide beneficiary access information on the program as a whole.

The results of CMS's beneficiary satisfaction survey were generally positive, although the survey had limitations. CMS obtained responses from at least 400 beneficiaries in each of the nine competitive bidding areas, and in each of nine non-CBP comparison markets—areas chosen to closely match the makeup of each of the competitive bidding areas. Responses were collected by telephone in these 18 locations both pre-CBP and post-CBP. The survey collected beneficiary satisfaction ratings on a five-point scale for six topic questions about the beneficiary's initial interaction with DME suppliers, the training received regarding the DME item, the delivery of the DME item, the quality of service provided by the supplier, the customer service provided by the supplier, and the supplier's overall complaint handling. Respondents answered these questions with one of five options from "very poor" to "very good."[79] Follow-up questions were not used to obtain more detailed information.

The survey design did not capture responses from beneficiaries living in those locations who may have needed, but did not obtain, DME during the period; that is, if a beneficiary's access problems resulted in his not receiving DME, that beneficiary would not be included in the survey. The survey's sampling methodology also did not ensure that all socio-economic groups were represented, so it does not confirm that all beneficiaries within an area had equal access.

---

[79]Respondents could also answer "not applicable."

CMS's beneficiary satisfaction survey did not reveal systemic beneficiary access or satisfaction problems with CBP. For all six questions in the competitive bidding areas, approximately 67 percent of beneficiaries reported their services as being "very good". Beneficiaries in competitive bidding areas rated as "good" or "very good" their initial interaction with the DME supplier (89 percent), the training received (86 percent), delivery (91 percent), quality (90 percent), customer service (88 percent), and complaint handling (84 percent). Results within competitive bidding areas show a drop of one to three percentage points on each of the six questions from pre-implementation to post-implementation. Beneficiaries in the comparison markets rated their experiences similarly to those in competitive bidding markets: these beneficiaries rated as "good" or "very good" their initial interaction with the DME supplier (93 percent), the training received (89 percent), delivery (93 percent), quality (93 percent), customer service (91 percent), and complaint handling (88 percent).

CMS's daily monitoring of national Medicare claims data in real time found no changes in health outcomes in competitive bidding areas in 2011, but this method may not fully capture the relationship between access to DME and health outcomes. CMS tracks health outcomes—such as hospitalizations, emergency room visits, physician visits, admissions to skilled nursing facilities, and deaths—for beneficiaries likely to use a CBP-covered product and who have used a CBP-covered product, in both competitive bidding areas and similar comparison areas. CMS reports that, in 2011, the rate of use of hospital services, emergency room visits, physician visits, and skilled nursing facility care for beneficiaries in competitive bidding areas remained consistent with national trends. While these results are reassuring, these measures do not show directly whether beneficiaries received the DME they needed on time, or whether health outcomes were caused by problems accessing CBP-covered DME.

In the first 6 months of 2011, CMS's online supplier locator tool may not have provided beneficiaries with up-to-date item availability for two reasons. First, CMS's update of its requirements after the second quarter no longer required suppliers to list the brands and models they had made available to beneficiaries in the previous quarter.[80] Therefore, CMS did not have records of supplies actually furnished, only of the type of supplies that contract suppliers intended to furnish. Second, suppliers we spoke with reported problems submitting the required forms in the first quarter of 2011, which may have caused a delay in updating information on the online supplier locator tool. These suppliers reported that the online submission form was unavailable during the period they were required to submit their first quarter data. They told us they had to submit hard copies of the forms, a time-consuming process which may have caused delays in reporting.

Early Data Indicate Some Decreases in DME Utilization

CMS data show that fewer distinct beneficiaries[81] in competitive bidding areas received CBP-covered DME items in 2011 than in 2010 for the six product categories that we analyzed.[82] However, we do not assume that the utilization in 2010 was the appropriate level of Medicare utilization and the decline in the number of beneficiaries served between 2010 and 2011 does not necessarily indicate that beneficiaries did not have access to needed DME. For example, the number of beneficiaries served in 2010 may have been inflated by suppliers billing for unnecessary items; and 2011 claims data may not yet be complete. Data on the utilization of mail-order diabetic testing supplies is limited because some beneficiaries used non-CBP retail suppliers.

---

[80]Initially, CMS required contract suppliers to submit a "form c" including information on both the brands supplied in the prior quarter and the brands they expected to furnish for the upcoming quarter. CMS issued a notice on September 28, 2011, stating that for the third quarter of 2011, contract suppliers only need to submit information on the brands and models they plan to offer during the next quarter, and are no longer required to provide information on items furnished during the previous quarter.

[81]Each distinct Medicare beneficiary is only counted once in each of the 6 months analyzed in 2010 and 2011 for each product category in a competitive bidding area, regardless of how many items that beneficiary received.

[82]We did not include these round 1 rebid product categories: (1) the mail-order diabetic testing supplies category due to some beneficiaries switching to non-mail order sources, a concern being studied by the HHS OIG; (2) the complex power wheelchair category due to potential data reliability concerns reported by a CMS contractor; and (3) the support surfaces category because it is limited to only the Miami competitive bidding area in the round 1 rebid.

Early Data Generally Indicate Utilization Decreases for Six CBP Product Categories

For the six CBP product categories we analyzed for CBP's first 6 months of 2011, initial Medicare claim data trends generally indicate a decrease in the number of CBP-covered Medicare beneficiaries who were furnished certain CBP-covered items.[83] The decrease is evident when comparing changes in the number of distinct CBP-covered beneficiaries served in 2011 compared to 2010 in both the nine competitive bidding areas and non-competitive bidding areas.[84] However, such decline in the number of beneficiaries served does not necessarily indicate beneficiaries do not have access to needed DME as CMS told us that possible reasons for the decline in utilization may be the result of:

- CBP's round 1 rebid competitive bidding areas were selected by CMS, in part because they had high utilization, implying that some utilization may have been unnecessary.

- CBP bidding requirements may have eliminated some suppliers that previously may have been involved in potentially fraudulent Medicare claims billing which could have inflated pre-CBP utilization. CBP Medicare claims can be more closely monitored for possible fraud because there are fewer suppliers furnishing items.

- Some suppliers may have increased their Medicare claims submissions prior to the CBP round 1 rebid's start date, which could have inflated 2010 utilization.

- Because suppliers have up to 1 year from the date of service to submit claims, the 2011 claims data may not yet be complete.

For the CPAP/RAD product category, the number of distinct CBP-covered beneficiaries who were furnished these items in the nine CBP competitive bidding areas was smaller in each of the first 6 months of 2011 than in the

---

[83]Medicare claims for the first 6 months of 2011 are based on data from claims processed as of February 17, 2012. Our analysis compares the change in the number of distinct Medicare beneficiaries furnished certain CBP-covered items in each product category—those among the top 34 HCPCS codes items that CMS determined represent the top 80 percent highest cost and highest utilization—in the nine competitive bidding areas and in non-competitive bidding areas. DME items included in our analysis are included in appendix I.

[84]Our analysis used the 2010 utilization data for comparison because it was the year immediately prior to CBP beginning in January 2011, and does not assume that 2010's utilization is the appropriate level for any of the CBP product categories.

same months of 2010. For example, in May 2010, 21,382 beneficiaries residing in the competitive bidding areas were furnished one or more CPAP/RAD product category items, while in May 2011, the number of beneficiaries furnished these items had declined by about 8 percent to 19,572. In contrast, in non-CBP competitive bidding areas, more beneficiaries were served in each of the first 6 months of 2011 compared to the same months in 2010. For example, in May 2010, 308,728 beneficiaries not residing in competitive bidding areas were furnished one or more CPAP/RAD product category items, while in May 2011, the number of beneficiaries furnished these items had risen to 333,746—for an increase of about 8 percent. (See fig. 8.)

Figure 8: Change in the Number of Distinct Medicare Beneficiaries Furnished Selected CBP-covered CPAP/RAD Product Category Items; Round 1 Rebid's First 6 Months 2011

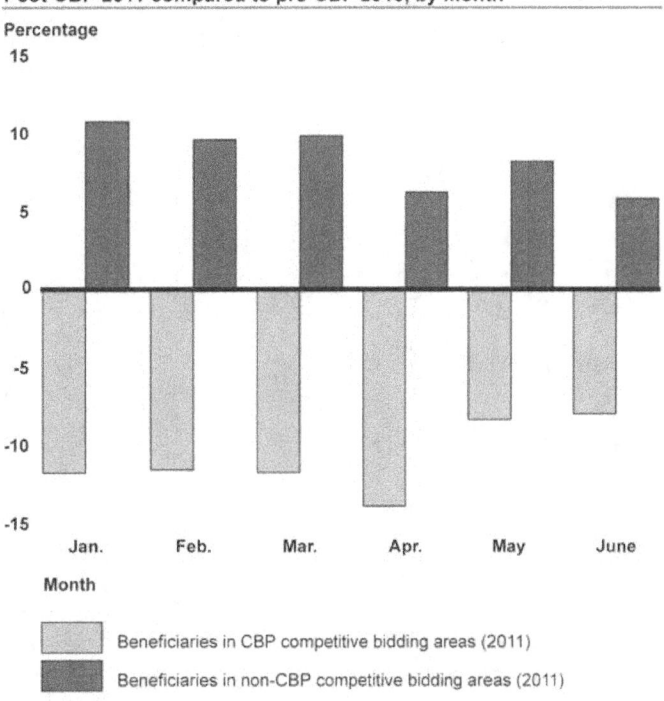

Post-CBP 2011 compared to pre-CBP 2010, by month

Percentage

Legend:
- Beneficiaries in CBP competitive bidding areas (2011)
- Beneficiaries in non-CBP competitive bidding areas (2011)

Source: GAO analysis of CMS data.

Notes: This analysis was based on Medicare claims data for the first 6 months of 2011, processed as of February 17, 2012. Our analysis is based on the 6 HCPCS codes related to this product category that are among the 34 HCPCS codes across all CBP product categories that CMS determined are the top 80 percent highest cost and highest utilization codes. (See appendix 1.)

For the enteral product category, there were fewer beneficiaries served in both the nine CBP competitive bidding areas and the non-competitive bidding areas in the first 6 months of 2011 compared to the same months of 2010. However, for every month between January and June, the number of beneficiaries served in competitive bidding areas showed a larger decrease from 2010 to 2011 than occurred in the same month for non-competitive bidding areas. For example, in May 2010, 5,378 beneficiaries residing in the competitive bidding areas were furnished one or more enteral product category items, while in May 2011, the number of beneficiaries furnished these items had decreased by almost 15 percent to 4,576. Similarly, in May 2010, 62,298 beneficiaries not residing in competitive bidding areas were furnished one or more enteral product category items, while in May 2011, the number of beneficiaries furnished these items decreased by about 9 percent to 56,680. Although both CBP competitive bidding areas and the non-competitive bidding areas showed a decrease in the number of beneficiaries served in May 2011 as compared to May 2010, the competitive bidding areas had an additional 6 percent decrease than the non-competitive bidding areas. (See fig.9.)

Figure 9: Change in the Number of Distinct Medicare Beneficiaries Furnished Selected CBP-covered Enteral Product Category Items; Round 1 Rebid's First 6 Months 2011

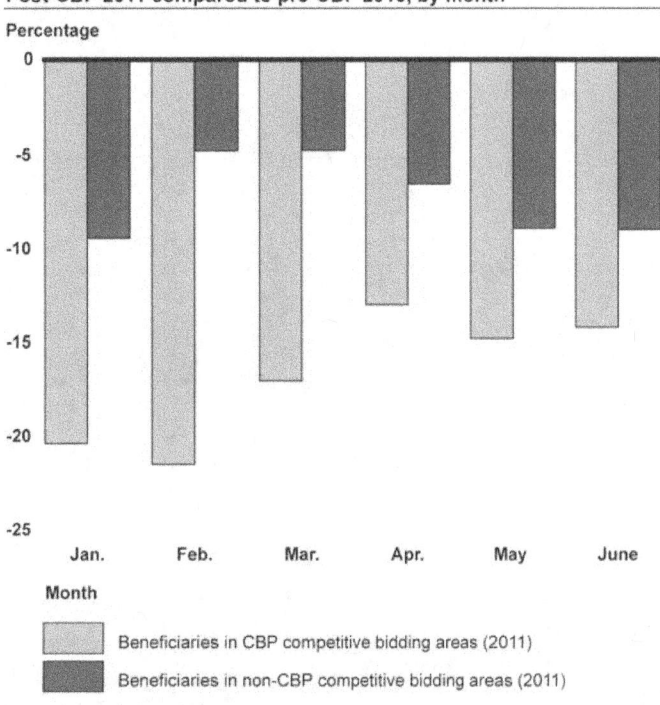

Post-CBP 2011 compared to pre-CBP 2010, by month

Source: GAO analysis of CMS data.

Notes: This analysis was based on Medicare claims data for the first 6 months of 2011, processed as of February 17, 2012. Our analysis is based on the 4 HCPCS codes related to this product category that are among the 34 HCPCS codes across all CBP product categories that CMS determined are the top 80 percent highest cost and highest utilization codes. (See appendix 1.)

For the hospital beds product category, the number of distinct CBP-covered beneficiaries who were served these items was smaller in each of the first 6 months of 2011 than in the same months of 2010. (See fig. 10.) In non-CBP competitive bidding areas, more beneficiaries were served in the first 3 months of 2011 than in the first 3 months of 2010 but progressively fewer beneficiaries were served in April, May, and June of 2011 than in the same months of 2010.

GAO-12-693 DME Competitive Bidding Program

Figure 10: Change in the Number of Distinct Medicare Beneficiaries Furnished Selected CBP-covered Hospital Bed Product Category Items; Round 1 Rebid's First 6 Months 2011

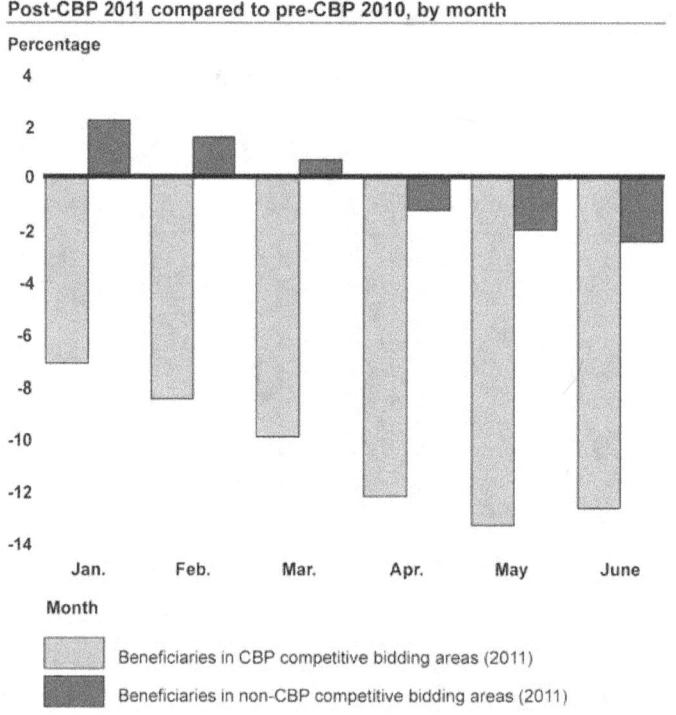

Post-CBP 2011 compared to pre-CBP 2010, by month

Source: GAO analysis of CMS data.

Notes: This analysis was based on Medicare claims data for the first 6 months of 2011, processed as of February 17, 2012. Our analysis is based on the 3 HCPCS codes related to this product category that are among the 34 HCPCS codes across all CBP product categories that CMS determined are the top 80 percent highest cost and highest utilization codes. (See appendix 1.)

For the oxygen product category, the number of distinct CBP-covered beneficiaries who were served these items in the nine CBP competitive bidding areas was smaller in each of the first 6 months of 2011 than in the same months of 2010. (See fig. 11.) Similar to what occurred for the hospital bed category, in non-CBP competitive bidding areas, more beneficiaries were served in the first 3 months of 2011 than in the first 3 months of 2010, but progressively fewer beneficiaries were served in April, May, and June of 2011 than in the same months of 2010.

Figure 11: Change in the Number of Distinct Medicare Beneficiaries Furnished Selected CBP-covered Oxygen Product Category Items; Round 1 Rebid's First 6 Months 2011

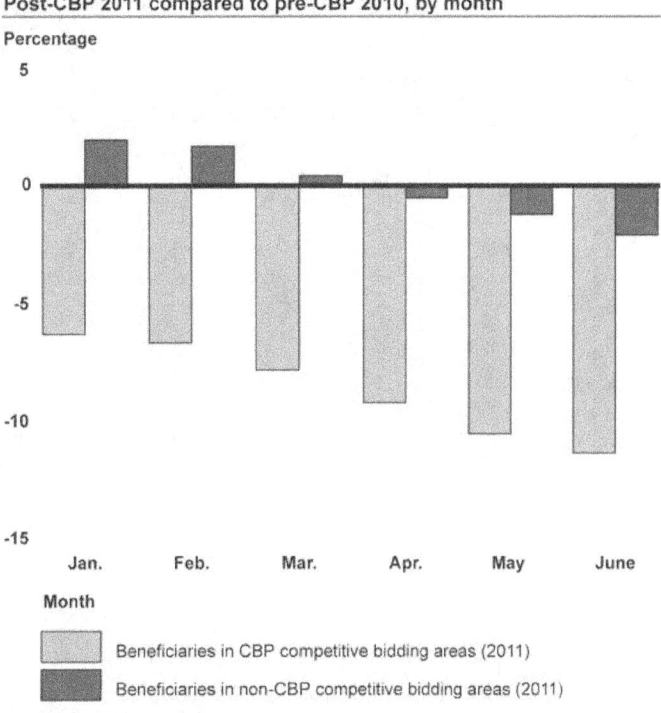

Post-CBP 2011 compared to pre-CBP 2010, by month

Percentage

Month

☐ Beneficiaries in CBP competitive bidding areas (2011)

■ Beneficiaries in non-CBP competitive bidding areas (2011)

Source: GAO analysis of CMS data.

Notes: This analysis was based on Medicare claims data for the first 6 months of 2011, processed as of February 17, 2012. Our analysis is based on the 6 HCPCS codes related to this product category that are among the 34 HCPCS codes across all CBP product categories that CMS determined are the top 80 percent highest cost and highest utilization codes. (See appendix 1.)

For the standard power wheelchair product category, the number of distinct CBP-covered beneficiaries who were served these items in the nine CBP competitive bidding areas was also smaller in the first 6 months of 2011 than in the same months of 2010.[85] While we included information about changes in utilization of the standard power wheelchair

---

[85]CMS told us that it found a noticeable spike in the number of standard power wheelchairs furnished in December 2010 for several competitive bidding areas. CMS said that there were 44 percent more claims in December 2010 than the average month in 2010 across all competitive bidding areas for this product category.

product category in competitive bidding areas, we did not include like information for non-competitive bidding areas because CMS changed the payment policy for standard power wheelchairs in non-competitive bidding areas only, making comparison to non-competitive bidding areas difficult. The payment policy change, effective January 1, 2011, eliminated the option for the lump sum purchase payment for standard power wheelchairs in all non-competitive bidding areas. (See fig. 12.) We also did not include utilization data for the complex wheelchair product category as it is unreliable due to suppliers' inconsistent use of Medicare claims payment modifiers.[86]

---

[86]Through its Pricing, Data Analysis and Coding Contractor-generated CBP monitoring reports, CMS has determined that some contract suppliers have been inconsistently using the Medicare claim payment modifiers for some items' HCPCS codes that are included in both the CBP standard and complex power wheelchair product categories. Because the two product categories have different CBP payments for the same items, the payment modifiers distinguish whether the item is for a standard or a complex power wheelchair.

Figure 12: Change in the Number of Distinct Medicare Beneficiaries Furnished Selected CBP-covered Standard Power Wheelchair Product Category Items; Round 1 Rebid's First 6 Months 2011

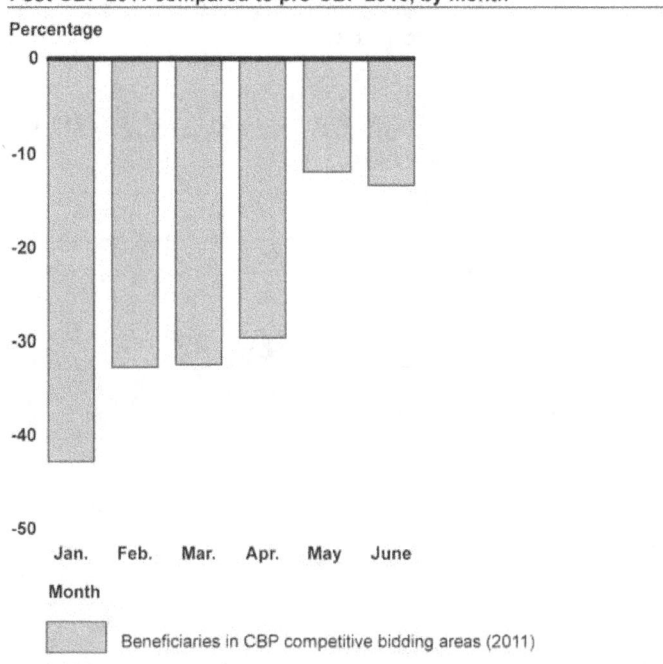

Post-CBP 2011 compared to pre-CBP 2010, by month

Source: GAO analysis of CMS data.

Notes: This analysis was based on Medicare claims data for the first 6 months of 2011, processed as of February 17, 2012. Our analysis is based on the 3 HCPCS codes related to this product category that are among the 34 HCPCS codes across all CBP product categories that CMS determined are the top 80 percent highest cost and highest utilization codes. (See appendix 1.)

For the walkers product category, the number of distinct CBP-covered beneficiaries who were furnished these items in the nine CBP competitive bidding areas was smaller in each of the first 6 months of 2011 than in the same months of 2010.[87] While more beneficiaries were served in non-CBP competitive bidding areas in January 2011 than in January 2010,

---

[87]CMS told us that the Medicare claims data for walkers may not capture a CBP exemption that allows physicians and other practitioners to furnish certain items, such as walkers, to their own patients as part of their professional service and hospitals to furnish certain items to the hospital's own patients during an admission or on the date of discharge.

fewer beneficiaries were served in February through June of 2011 compared to the same months of 2010. (See fig. 13.)

Figure 13: Change in the Number of Distinct Medicare Beneficiaries Furnished Selected CBP-covered Walkers Product Category Items; Round 1 Rebid's First 6 Months 2011

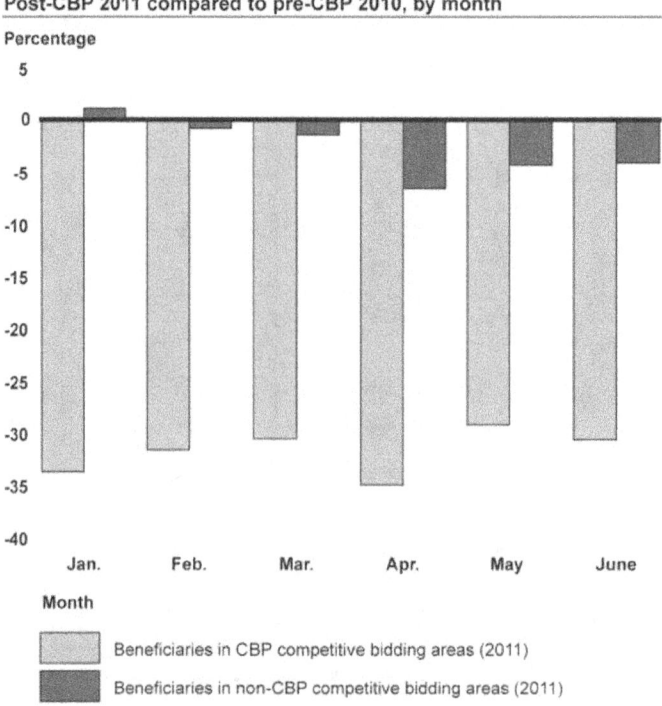

Post-CBP 2011 compared to pre-CBP 2010, by month

Source: GAO analysis of CMS data.

Notes: This analysis was based on Medicare claims data for the first 6 months of 2011, processed as of February 17, 2012. Our analysis is based on the 3 HCPCS codes related to this product category that are among the 34 HCPCS codes across all CBP product categories that CMS determined are the top 80 percent highest cost and highest utilization codes. (See appendix 1.)

CBP's Mail-order Diabetic Testing Supplies Utilization Data Affected by Some CBP-covered Beneficiaries Choosing Higher Cost Non-CBP Non-mail-order Retail Suppliers

Although CBP-covered beneficiaries pay less for their diabetic testing supplies if they choose a CBP mail-order contract supplier, CMS has determined that some CBP-covered beneficiaries who had been receiving their supplies by mail-order in 2010 have been switching to non-mail-order sources in 2011. This switching would decrease both CBP's mail-order utilization and its anticipated Medicare savings.

CBP's diabetic testing supplies product category is the only category that allows CBP-covered beneficiaries to choose how to receive their supplies—delivered by mail-order from a CBP contract supplier or furnished by a non-mail-order retail or storefront supplier. The beneficiary's choice determines whether the CBP-covered supplies are paid at the CBP single payment amounts or at the Medicare fee schedule payments, and whether the beneficiary's coinsurance is based on the lower CBP payment or the higher fee schedule payment.

The HHS OIG is studying the extent to which and why beneficiaries have switched from mail-order to non-mail-order suppliers between 2010 (the year prior to CBP) and 2011 (the first year of CBP).[88] There are concerns that suppliers may be providing testing supplies by mail-order but billing at the non-mail-order fee schedule payments, or may be incentivizing beneficiaries to choose non-mail-order instead of mail-order. The HHS OIG has stated that either of these activities could affect CBP mail-order utilization and projected CBP Medicare savings.

---

[88]In order to not duplicate efforts, we consulted with the HHS OIG about its work and agreed to focus our work on the aggregate CBP mail-order utilization. Since these data are affected by beneficiaries switching from mail or non-mail-order, and the reasons for the switching are being studied by the OIG, we determined that, at this point in the CBP, the utilization data were unreliable for our purposes.

Both CMS and DME Suppliers Incurred Costs During the CBP Round 1 Rebid, but CMS Estimates Significant Medicare Savings

Both CMS and suppliers incurred costs related to CBP. However, CMS estimates that CBP savings to Medicare and to beneficiaries are greater than its costs.

CMS Reported Costs of Nearly $20 Million in the 18 Months Prior to the Round 1 Rebid Start, and Contract Suppliers Reported Varying Costs to Participate

CMS told us that it spent nearly $20 million on pre-implementation costs for the CBP round 1 rebid from May 2009 through December 2010. In August 2009, CMS began the suppliers' bidding education campaign, and the round 1 rebid bid window opened on October 21, 2009. The CBP costs incurred during this time included outreach materials for beneficiaries, referral agents, and others, an IT contract, and other implementation costs. (See table 10.)

Table 10: CMS Operational Costs for CBP, May 2009 through December 2010

Cost description	Cost to CMS	Percentage of total cost
Palmetto GBA contract to implement CBP	$11,466,333	58.24%
CMS CBP-related administrative costs[a]	3,002,000	15.25
Public outreach materials related to CBP	2,516,294	12.78
IT contract for CBP bid submission system[b]	1,597,614	8.11
CAO and office to respond to CBP-related questions and complaints[c]	1,000,666	5.08
PAOC meetings[d]	105,000	0.53
Total	**$19,687,907**	**100**

Source: GAO analysis of information provided by CMS.

Notes: This table does not include training and salaries for 1-800-MEDICARE phone workers, script answer development, or CMS regional office caseworkers. While CMS trained CSRs to respond solely to CBP-related calls, CMS did not provide cost information for these CSRs.

[a]CMS's internal administrative costs include 12 CMS staff that primarily work on CBP in the Division of DMEPOS Policy or the Division of DMEPOS Competitive Bidding, using average salary and other employment costs of $158,000 per employee.

[b]CMS developed the Durable Medical Equipment, Prosthetics, Orthotics, and Supplies bidding system (DBidS) to correct the operational problems identified in the previous system.

[c]Costs for the CAO and her office include four employees using average salary and other employment costs of $158,000 per employee.

[d]PAOC members are appointed by the HHS Secretary to advise CMS on implementing the CBP. One PAOC meeting was held during this time period on April 5, 2011.

In its 2007 CBP Final Rule, CMS estimated that a bidding supplier spends an average of $2,303.16 to prepare bids for CBP, and in May 2011, CMS officials told us that this estimate had not changed. Suppliers and supplier organizations told us they incurred varying costs when preparing a bid, including fees for legal and financial services. For example, one supplier hired a new staff member to oversee the bidding process, and some suppliers reported paying for assistance in compiling the required financial documentation. Some suppliers reported additional legal services to prepare their bids.

Contract suppliers also incurred expenses for participating in the program. Winning suppliers may incur additional expenses to fulfill their contractual obligations—for example, one supplier told us that it paid up to $1,500 for updates to a software program in order to provide CMS the data required under CBP. Suppliers that subcontract with contract suppliers stated that they also incur expenses, such as the costs involved in negotiating an agreement with the contract supplier.

CMS Estimates that CBP Round 1 Rebid Will Result in Significant Savings for Both the Medicare Program and Beneficiaries

CMS's estimated savings to both the Medicare program and beneficiaries is significantly higher than its costs. In a 2012 report,[89] CMS estimated the CBP saved Medicare approximately $202.1 million in its first year of implementation, a decrease in expenditures of over 42 percent in the nine competitive bidding areas. This estimate is larger than the CMS's 2011 estimate, which did not include possible reductions in claims due to a decline in utilization. According to CMS, most savings come from the oxygen, mail-order diabetic supplies, and standard power wheelchair product categories. CMS also reported that CBP resulted in savings for beneficiaries.

Agency Comments and Our Evaluation

HHS reviewed a draft of this report and provided written comments which are reprinted in appendix II. HHS also provided technical comments, which we incorporated as appropriate.

---

[89]CMS's April 17, 2012 Competitive Bidding One Year Implementation Update can be found at http://www.cms.gov/MEDICARE/MEDICARE-FEE-FOR-SERVICE-PAYMENT/ DMEPOSCOMPETITIVEBID/INDEX.HTML.

HHS made several general comments. First, HHS noted that the CBP round 1 rebid resulted in savings of more than $200 million in its first year, and that the Department anticipates additional savings of more than $25 billion to the Medicare program between 2013 and 2022 as CBP expands in round 2. Second, HHS commented that we had not fully accounted for the robust nature of CMS's real-time claims monitoring system that measures the health status of Medicare beneficiaries using DME in both CBP and comparison areas, which HHS said indicates that CBP-covered beneficiaries have not been adversely affected by CBP . We revised the report to incorporate more details about the monitoring program, but we believe that our original description of the program was accurate. We concluded that, in the aggregate, CMS's monitoring efforts provide useful information about beneficiary access and satisfaction. Third, HHS stated that we agreed with its view that the CBP round 1 rebid had reduced unnecessary utilization of DME. We noted that the CBP may have successfully reduced unnecessary DME utilization, because utilization has been reduced and CMS has not detected adverse health consequences, but our analysis does not allow us to conclude definitively that unnecessary utilization has been reduced. Moreover, we concluded that more experience with DME competitive bidding is needed to assess the program's full effects. Fourth, HHS suggested that January 2011 was not an appropriate month to use in our examples of utilization changes associated with the round 1 rebid because it was the first month of the rebid. We agree and have changed our examples to May 2011.

Finally, HHS discussed differences between CMS's methods for measuring DME utilization changes associated with the CBP and our methodology, and noted disparities between CMS's results and our findings. HHS noted that CMS monitors all DME claims in real-time in both CBP and matched comparison areas, and that its analyses are comparisons between the types of areas. As HHS noted, we analyzed claims data for DME items accounting for 80 percent of DME costs and utilization, not all items. We compared DME utilization in CBP round 1 rebid areas to the rest of the country, not to specific comparator areas. In addition, we analyzed claims for services provided in the months January through June in 2011 and compared them to the same months in 2010. Because the process of filing and processing Medicare claims can be lengthy, we used data for claims that had been processed by CMS's payment contractors as of February 2012. We believe that our methods are valid. Further, our results are similar to results that CMS reported to us in its technical comments. For example, CMS found that 14 percent fewer beneficiaries had claims for hospital bed product category items in CBP areas in 2011 than in 2010. We found that about 13 percent fewer

GAO-12-693 DME Competitive Bidding Program

beneficiaries had claims for these items in May 2011 than in May 2010 in the CBP areas.

Concluding Observations

Although the first year of the CBP round 1 rebid's contracts has been completed, it is important to continue to closely monitor the CBP as the program expands into 91 additional areas in round 2. Our findings are based on the limited evidence available at the time we did our work. It is too soon to determine the full effects the CBP may have on Medicare beneficiaries and DME suppliers.

We found that, in general, the round 1 rebid was successfully implemented. Nearly the same number of suppliers participated in the round 1 rebid as in CBP round 1. Few contract suppliers left Medicare during CBP's first year. CMS's beneficiary satisfaction survey and other monitoring activities, although limited, does not show evidence that beneficiaries have been affected negatively by CBP. Utilization of selected DME items declined in the round 1 rebid competitive bidding areas; however, we do not assume that all pre-CBP utilization was appropriate and CBP may have reduced unnecessary utilization of DME, particularly because CMS chose to implement the CBP round 1 rebid in areas with what it suspected were relatively high levels of unnecessary utilization.

More experience with DME competitive bidding is needed, particularly to see if evidence of beneficiary access problems emerges. In the program's first year, the prevalence of grandfathered suppliers for rental items may have ameliorated beneficiary access concerns. The number of grandfathered suppliers will continue to decrease as rental periods expire. Further, it is not known if the number of subcontracting suppliers will remain consistent or whether any change in subcontracting may affect beneficiary access to DME. While few contract suppliers voluntarily withdrew from CBP or were terminated by CMS in the first contract year, an increase in either outcome throughout the remaining contract period could have implications for beneficiary access and the CBP itself. Additionally, it will be important to determine if DME utilization trends similar to those in the round 1 rebid occur as the program expands into round 2's competitive bidding areas.

We are sending copies of this report to the Secretary of Health and Human Services. The report will also be available at no charge on our website at http://www.gao.gov.

If you or your staffs have any questions about this report, please contact me at (202) 512-7114 or kingk@gao.gov. Contact points for our Offices of Congressional Relations and Public Affairs may be found on the last page of this report. GAO staff who made major contributions to this report are listed in appendix III.

Kathleen M. King
Director, Health Care

Appendix I: HCPCS Codes that CMS Determined Are the Top 80 Percent Highest Cost and Utilization for CBP Round 1 Rebid

Product Category	HCPCS Code	Description
Complex Rehabilitative Power Wheelchairs and Related Accessories (Group 2)	K0835	Power wheelchair, group 2 standard, single power option, sling/solid seat/back, patient weight capacity up to and including 300 pounds
	K0836	Power wheelchair, group 2 standard, single power option, captains chair, patient weight capacity up to and including 300 pounds
	K0843	Power wheelchair, group 2 heavy duty, multiple power option, sling/solid seat/back, patient weight capacity 301 to 450 pounds
Continuous Positive Airway Pressure Devices, Respiratory Assist Devices, and Related Supplies and Accessories (CPAP/RAD)	A7030	Full face mask used with positive airway pressure device (each)
	A7034	Nasal interface (mask or cannula type) used with positive airway pressure device, with or without head strap
	A7037	Tubing used with positive airway pressure device
	E0470	Respiratory assist device, bi-level pressure capability, without backup rate feature, used with noninvasive interface, e.g., nasal or facial mask (intermittent assist device with continuous positive airway pressure device)
	E0562	Humidifier, heated, used with positive airway pressure device
	E0601	Continuous airway pressure (CPAP) device
Enteral Nutrients, Equipment, and Supplies	B4035	Enteral feeding supply kit; pump fed, per day; includes but not limited to feeding/flushing syringe, administration set tubing, dressings, tape
	B4150	Enteral formula, nutritionally complete with intact nutrients, includes proteins, fats, carbohydrates, vitamins and minerals, may include fiber, administered through an enteral feeding tube, 100 calories =1 unit
	B4152	Enteral formula, nutritionally complete, calorically dense (equal to or greater than 1.5 kcal/ml) with intact nutrients, includes proteins, fats, carbohydrates, vitamins and minerals, may Include fiber, administered through an enteral feeding tube, 100 calories =1 unit
	B4154	Enteral formula, nutritionally complete, for special metabolic needs, excludes inherited disease of metabolism, includes altered composition of proteins, fats, carbohydrates, vitamins and/or minerals, may include fiber, administered through an enteral feeding tube, 100 calories =1 unit
Hospital Beds and Related Accessories	E0260	Hospital bed, semi-electric (head and foot adjustment), with any type side rails, with mattress
	E0261	Hospital bed, semi-electric (head and foot adjustment), with any type side rails, without mattress
	E0303	Hospital bed, heavy duty, extra wide, with weight capacity greater than 350 pounds, but less than or equal to 600 pounds, with any type side rails, with mattress
Mail-Order Diabetic Supplies[a]	A4253	Blood glucose test or reagent strips for home blood glucose monitor, per 50 strips: item delivered via mail
	A4259	Lancets, per box of 100: item delivered via mail
	A4256	Normal, low and high calibrator solution/chips: item delivered via mail

Product Category	HCPCS Code	Description
Oxygen Supplies and Equipment	E0424	Stationary compressed gaseous oxygen system, rental; includes container, contents, regulator, flowmeter, humidifier, nebulizer, cannula or mask, and tubing
	E0439	Stationary liquid oxygen system, rental; includes container, contents, regulator, flowmeter, humidifier, nebulizer, cannula or mask, and tubing
	E1390	Oxygen concentrator, single delivery port, capable of delivering 85 percent or greater oxygen concentration at the prescribed flow rate
	E1391	Oxygen concentrator, dual delivery port, capable of delivering 85 percent or greater oxygen concentration at the prescribed flow rate (each)
	E0431	Portable gaseous oxygen system, rental; includes portable container, regulator, flowmeter, humidifier, cannula or mask, and tubing
	E0434	Portable liquid oxygen system, rental; includes portable container, supply reservoir, humidifier, flowmeter, refill adaptor, contents gauge, cannula or mask, and tubing
Standard Power Wheelchairs, Scooters, and Related Accessories	K0823	Power wheelchair, group 2 standard, captains chair, patient weight capacity up to and including 300 pounds
	K0822	Power wheelchair, group 2 standard, sling/solid seat/back, patient weight capacity up to and including 300 pounds
	K0825	Power wheelchair, group 2 heavy duty, captains chair, patient weight capacity 301 to 450 pounds
Support Surfaces (Group 2 Mattresses and Overlays)	E0277	Powered pressure reducing air mattress
	E0372	Powered air overlay for mattress, standard mattress length and width
	E0373	Non-powered advanced pressure reducing mattress
Walkers and Related Accessories	E0135	Walker, folding (pickup), adjustable or fixed height
	E0143	Walker, folding, wheeled, adjustable or fixed height
	E0156	Seat attachment, walker

Source: GAO analysis of CMS and Palmetto GBA information.

[a]The three HCPCS codes under the mail-order diabetic supplies product category must also include the modifier "KL" at the end to indicate that these supplies were furnished by mail-order.

Appendix II: Comments from the Department of Health and Human Services

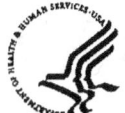

DEPARTMENT OF HEALTH & HUMAN SERVICES

OFFICE OF THE SECRETARY

Assistant Secretary for Legislation
Washington, DC 20201

MAY 08 2012

Kathleen King
Director, Health Care
U.S. Government Accountability Office
441 G Street NW
Washington, DC 20548

Dear Ms. King:

Attached are comments on the U.S. Government Accountability Office's (GAO) report entitled: "MEDICARE: Review of the First Year of CMS's Durable Medical Equipment Competitive Bidding Program's Round 1 Rebid" (GAO-12-693).

The Department appreciates the opportunity to review this draft section of the report prior to publication.

Sincerely,

Jim R. Esquea
Assistant Secretary for Legislation

Attachment

<u>**GENERAL COMMENTS OF THE DEPARTMENT OF HEALTH AND HUMAN
SERVICES (HHS) ON THE GOVERNMENT ACCOUNTABILITY OFFICE'S (GAO)
DRAFT REPORT ENTITLED, "MEDICARE: REVIEW OF THE FIRST YEAR OF
CMS'S DURABLE MEDICAL EQUIPMENT COMPETITIVE BIDDING PROGRAMS'S
ROUND 1 REBID" (GAO-12-693)**</u>

The Department appreciates the opportunity to review and comment on this draft report.

The Department recently released a report documenting the Medicare Durable Medical
Equipment, Prosthetics, Orthotics, and Supplies (DMEPOS) Competitive Bidding Program's
first year results, which include savings to Medicare of approximately $202.1 million and
preservation of beneficiary access and health status outcomes.[1] We are pleased that the GAO
also found that the program was implemented successfully.

As briefly mentioned in the draft report, CMS implemented a variety of operational
improvements to the program prior to the Round 1 Rebid based on statutory changes, an
evaluation of the 2008 bidding process, feedback from stakeholders, and advice from the
Program Advisory and Oversight Committee for the Competitive Acquisition Program. Some
examples of these key operational improvements include: a process under which suppliers could
qualify to be notified of missing financial bid documents; an upgraded bidder education program
completed prior to the opening of the bid window; a new and improved online bidding system;
and enhanced bid evaluation processes such as a comprehensive upfront licensing verification
process; a more rigorous bona fide bid evaluation process; and increased scrutiny of expansion
plans for suppliers new to an area or product category. We believe these operational
modifications to the program resulted in a bidding process that was easier for suppliers to
navigate and that ultimately benefitted Medicare beneficiaries.

While we appreciate GAO's general findings of successful implementation, we believe that the
GAO analysis did not fully account for the robustness of CMS's real-time claims monitoring
system. This sophisticated new system analyzes 100 percent of Medicare claims using over
3,400 indicators, including potential changes in key secondary indicators such as hospital
admissions, emergency room visits, physician visits, and admissions to skilled nursing facilities
before and after the implementation of the new payment model. The monitoring system looks at
three comparison groups of beneficiaries over time: 1) all Medicare beneficiaries living in one of
the nine areas compared to beneficiaries living in a similar geographic area not yet subject to
competitive bidding (e.g., Orlando vs. Tampa); 2) beneficiaries in one of the nine areas most
likely to use a particular item compared to beneficiaries in a similar geographic area most likely
to use the item; and 3) beneficiaries actually using an item living in one of the nine areas
compared to beneficiaries actually using an item living in a similar geographic area.

---

[1]*Competitive Bidding Update—One Year Implementation Update*, April 17, 2012.
http://www.cms.gov/Medicare/Medicare-Fee-for-Service-
Payment/DMEPOSCompetitiveBid/Downloads/Competitive-Bidding-Update-One-Year-Implementation.pdf

1

<u>**GENERAL COMMENTS OF THE DEPARTMENT OF HEALTH AND HUMAN
SERVICES (HHS) ON THE GOVERNMENT ACCOUNTABILITY OFFICE'S (GAO)
DRAFT REPORT ENTITLED, "MEDICARE: REVIEW OF THE FIRST YEAR OF
CMS'S DURABLE MEDICAL EQUIPMENT COMPETITIVE BIDDING PROGRAMS'S
ROUND 1 REBID" (GAO-12-693)**</u>

The real-time claims monitoring system has consistently demonstrated that there have been no
changes to beneficiary health status outcomes resulting from the competitive bidding program.[2]
For example, the rate of use of hospital services, emergency room visits, physician visits, and
skilled nursing facility care in competitive bidding areas has remained consistent with the
patterns and trends seen throughout the rest of the country. CMS has also used this system to
monitor utilization of DMEPOS and follow up with additional investigation as needed. For
example, monitoring revealed declines in the use of mail-order diabetes test strips and
continuous positive airway pressure supplies in the competitive bidding areas. In response to
these declines, CMS conducted outreach to beneficiaries with claims in 2010. CMS found that,
in virtually every case, the beneficiary reported having more than enough supplies on hand, often
multiple months worth, and therefore, did not need to obtain additional supplies when the
program began.

HHS agrees with GAO's finding that the program curbed unnecessary utilization. We believe
GAO's analysis in this regard could have been enhanced through use of CMS real-time claims
monitoring data. For example, by examining trends over time and comparing changes in
competitive bidding areas to comparable areas, CMS found spikes in claims submission that
occurred immediately before program implementation. CMS also found that declines in
utilization were often more common in fraud-prone areas. Both of these findings provide further
evidence that beneficiary access to medically necessary items has been preserved under
the program.

As indicated in the draft report, the DMEPOS competitive bidding program will expand
substantially in 2013 with the implementation of Round 2 and the National Mail-Order Program
to furnish diabetic testing supplies. This expansion is expected to yield significant savings for
taxpayers and Medicare beneficiaries. CMS estimates that the program will save the Medicare
Part B Trust Fund $25.7 billion and beneficiaries $17.1 billion between 2013 and 2022. CMS
will continue to monitor the program carefully through all phases of implementation to ensure
that Medicare savings are achieved without negative consequences to Medicare beneficiaries.

HHS is concerned that the description of CMS's real-time claims monitoring system does not
accurately convey the sophistication, robustness, and usefulness of this new system to track and
prevent any potential problems for patients. We believe this should be reevaluated in the final
report. We would be pleased to provide a briefing to explain this system in more detail.

---

[2] Examples of real-time claims monitoring tracking can be found on the CMS website at:
http://www.cms.gov/Medicare/Medicare-Fee-for-Service-Payment/DMEPOSCompetitiveBid/Monitoring.html

2

GENERAL COMMENTS OF THE DEPARTMENT OF HEALTH AND HUMAN
SERVICES (HHS) ON THE GOVERNMENT ACCOUNTABILITY OFFICE'S (GAO)
DRAFT REPORT ENTITLED, "MEDICARE: REVIEW OF THE FIRST YEAR OF
CMS'S DURABLE MEDICAL EQUIPMENT COMPETITIVE BIDDING PROGRAMS'S
ROUND 1 REBID" (GAO-12-693)

Finally, HHS has compared the utilization figures in the draft report to real time-claims
monitoring system data and has the following comments:

- GAO included several specific counts that do not directly track with the monitoring data
  we are reviewing internally. There are disparities between GAO's utilization data
  compared to the real-time claims monitoring data used by CMS for internal review.

- GAO restricted its analyses to the top 80 percent of HCPCS over six months, whereas
  CMS observed all claims longitudinally from 2008 through 2011. Our methodologies
  also differed with respect to CMS' use of comparison regions, versus GAO's
  comparisons to nationally observed data. Finally, while not clear from the report, it is
  also possible that GAO and CMS applied different methodologies to the assignment of
  claims to specific beneficiary months, or to the use of paid versus unpaid claims.

- GAO frequently cites January 2011 data in this report. We believe the focus on January
  2011 data casts a misleading story with respect to utilization, since we observed increased
  utilization for several product categories and in several Competitive Bidding Areas'
  (CBAs) prior to the start of the Competitive Bidding Program (CBP).

- GAO identified several product categories that experienced a decrease in utilization. We
  have conducted a detailed analysis of declines in utilization, and we identified that
  decreases in utilization were frequently more prominent in one or two CBAs. As GAO
  correctly states, 2010 utilization data for CBAs may have been elevated due to
  inappropriate utilization of CBP products and supplies.

- CMS generally compares utilization and health outcomes for CBAs to comparator
  regions, rather than the rest of the nation. CMS identified comparator regions based on
  regional and demographic similarities which may or may not be present in a national
  cohort. Despite some changes in utilization, we have observed no changes in health
  outcomes in the total population, beneficiaries actually using competitively bid items, or
  in access groups of beneficiaries more likely to use competitively bid products.

3

Appendix III: GAO Contact and Staff Acknowledgments

GAO Contact	Kathleen M. King, (202) 512-7114 or kingk@gao.gov
Staff Acknowledgments	In addition to the contact named above, key contributors to this report were Martin T. Gahart, Assistant Director; Krister Friday, Dan Lee, Lisa Motley, Michelle Paluga, Katherine Perry, Hemi Tewarson, and Opal Winebrenner.

Related GAO Products

Medicare: Issues for Manufacturer-level Competitive Bidding for Durable Medical Equipment, GAO-11-337R. Washington, D.C.: May 31, 2011.

Medicare: CMS Has Addressed Some Implementation Problems from Round 1 of the Durable Medical Equipment Competitive Bidding Program for the Round 1 Rebid, GAO-10-1057T. Washington, D.C.: September 15, 2010.

Medicare: CMS Working to Address Problems from Round 1 of the Durable Medical Equipment Competitive Bidding Program. GAO-10-27. Washington, D.C.: November 6, 2009.

Medicare: Covert Testing Exposes Weaknesses in the Durable Medical Equipment Supplier Screening Process. GAO-08-955. Washington, D.C.: July 3, 2008.

Medicare: Competitive Bidding for Medical Equipment and Supplies Could Reduce Program Payments, but Adequate Oversight Is Critical. GAO-08-767T. Washington, D.C.: May 6, 2008.

Medicare: Improvements Needed to Address Improper Payments for Medical Equipment and Supplies. GAO-07-59. Washington, D.C.: January 31, 2007.

Medicare Payment: CMS Methodology Adequate to Estimate National Error Rate. GAO-06-300. Washington, D.C.: March 24, 2006.

Medicare Durable Medical Equipment: Class III Devices Do Not Warrant a Distinct Annual Payment Update. GAO-06-62. Washington, D.C.: March 1, 2006.

Medicare: More Effective Screening and Stronger Enrollment Standards Needed for Medical Equipment Suppliers. GAO-05-656. Washington, D.C.: September 22, 2005.

Medicare: CMS's Program Safeguards Did Not Deter Growth in Spending for Power Wheelchairs. GAO-05-43. Washington, D.C.: November 17, 2004.

Medicare: Past Experience Can Guide Future Competitive Bidding for Medical Equipment and Supplies. GAO-04-765. Washington, D.C.: September 7, 2004.

Medicare: CMS Did Not Control Rising Power Wheelchair Spending. GAO-04-716T. Washington, D.C.: April 28, 2004.